SURVIVING THE STROKE

A Minute with God

A Recovery and Rehabilitation Guide

Marty Martin

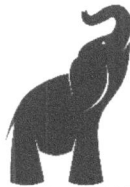

Little Elephant Publishing

For more information contact:
survivingthestroke.com/
info@martymartin.net
Martymartin.net

ISBN - Paperback: 978-1-955129-48-0
ISBN - Ebook: 978-1-955129-46-6
ISBN - Audiobook: 978-1-955129-47-3

Cover design by Marty Martin
Interior Design by Kindlepreneur
https://kindlepreneur.com/book-formatting/

First Edition: January 2025

CONTENTS

DEDICATION

Dedicated to Debbie Kay, my forever and supportive partner and wife who took care of me and tolerated me during the stroke and rehabilitation experience. To all my kids and grandkids for their love and support. They all pitched in and demonstrated what family is all about.

The Family: Debbie Kay, Shelby, Jessica, Buddy, Tanya, Joe, and the grandkids, Dean, Levi, Mirielle, and we cannot leave out our grey blue-eyed Boston terrier, Izzie.

ACKNOWLEDGEMENTS

Special thanks to everyone involved in my stroke event, recovery, and rehabilitation, beginning with the Ambulance crew from the Creve Coeur Fire Department, the ER and ICU team at Mercy Hospital St. Louis, and Dr. Thorley, Dr. Cotterell, and the entire staff at Mercy Rehabilitation Hospital. Also extra thanks to my neurologist, Dr. Jeffrey Calvin, and my primary physician, Dr. Karl Taria.

A very special thanks to the staff at the SSM Health Day Institute, otherwise known as Outpatient Therapy, in Chesterfield, Missouri, who guided me through ten months of recovery and rehabilitation.

One more special thanks goes to Barb, my trainer at GYMGUYZ.

One last special thanks must to go to my family, who were fully involved in my recovery and rehabilitation and provided all the extra care that was needed.

FOREWARD

Stroke is a devastating condition, not just for the victims of stroke themselves, but also for family members of the afflicted, and indeed for their entire community.

Recovery from stroke is often a long and difficult road, fraught with physical, emotional, and psychological ups and downs. It is not a smooth or easy process. Many stroke survivors must learn to adapt and take new approaches to everyday problems.

In sharing his personal story, Marty seeks to empower other stroke survivors and their families to navigate the rehabilitation journey.

Jeffrey S. Calvin, MD

Dr. Jeffrey Calvin is certified in neurology and clinical neurophysiology by the American Board of Psychiatry and Neurology. He is affiliated with Mercy Hospital of St. Louis and attended medical school at Rosalind Franklin University of Medicine and Science in Chicago. He went on to a neurology residence and clinical neurophysiology fellowship at Saint Louis University.

INTRODUCTION

Is This Book for You?

If you recently had a moderate to severe stroke or you are a caretaker for someone who had a stroke, I'd say yes, this book is for you. However, I will add that it all depends on the severity of the stroke or other serious injury resulting in hospitalization and partial paralysis. My experience was a month in the hospital followed by ten months attending outpatient therapy; therefore, my stroke would be considered moderate to severe. I've combined my personal experience with what I believe would be a useful how-to and what-to-expect guide. All the professionals who cared for me were excellent. I have no complaints there. However, while I was in the hospital, I felt that some sort of firsthand experience guide would have been helpful in preparing myself and my family for what was next, and so here we are: I wrote a book that I hope will provide both the victim and their families insight as to what's ahead.

During my months in outpatient therapy, the majority of patients were stroke victims—probably about 80% of them. The other patients were there due to work accidents, car accidents, diving accidents, ladder falls, neurological issues, COVID, surgery-related, or unknown causes of varying stages of paralysis. If you are a spouse, partner, or a caretaker for someone who has experienced these events, you'll also find information and insights to prepare you.

My intention for writing this book is to provide stroke or injury victims and their family and caretakers with a simple guide from someone with the actual personal experience of the recovery and rehabilitation process. My hope is that I can provide guidance and inspiration to help others navigate through the journey ahead and share insights that I have learned during my recovery process that will make your journey a bit less difficult, less stressful, and more productive.

If I have helped just one person navigate their stroke experience, then I've accomplished what I set out to do.

You've Had a Stroke and Survived...Now What?

On March 14, 2022, I had a hemorrhagic stroke. The majority of strokes occur in people who are 65 or older. It is estimated that 10% of people in the U.S. who experience a stroke are younger than 45. In the United States, about 795,000 people suffer a stroke each year (UTMB Health 2024). It is sad to think about, but most everyone has known or will know someone who had a stroke.

If you are reading this or listening to the audio version, you've either had a stroke or you know someone who's had a stroke. You may also have suffered a spinal injury, a fall, some other sort of serious injury, or an unexplained condition such as hemiplegia that can cause the same paralyzing symptoms as a stroke.

The hemorrhagic stroke I suffered was considered severe versus a mini or mild stroke. Through that experience, I discovered there was a lot happening and would continue to happen in the coming weeks and months. As the days passed, very good information was provided by the medical professionals. However, I found a lack of information preparing me for actual experiences of what would come next. Please do not misunderstand: The doctors and staff were great at explaining what was happening, and there are a lot of resources available, but it did not provide specific relatable experiences concerning recovery and rehabilitation.

Navigating and working through the recovery process requires a positive attitude, and having a sense of humor at times can help and even be therapeutic during recovery. Therefore, you may on occasion be exposed to my attempt at humor, including my references to movies and use of analogies.

If you happen to be listening to the audio version, you will notice the British accent, and sorry to disappoint, I am not British. I'm American and grew up in New York City and now live in the St. Louis, Missouri, area, but I thought a British accent would have a nice ring to it, and there you go—humor.

A Ridiculous Task

I say a ridiculous task because asking someone to read a book after a stroke may seem like a ridiculous suggestion. However, had someone given me this type of book or audiobook within my first few days, I believe things would have been a bit easier and prepared me and my family a little better, or at the very least, we would have known what to expect next. It's fully understandable that it may not be possible or desirable to read a book after a stroke but reading or listening as soon as possible is important because there is so much information that you will be exposed to, and a lot of it may not necessarily prepare you for all the aspects of recovery, such as the little things that you will be experiencing. It's easy to tell someone to read a book; however, if your vision has been impacted by a stroke, reading may not be an option, whereas an audiobook will work, especially with the help of a lovely British accent.

One thing about stroke victims is while we are all similar, we have different levels of what the stroke has done to us. For some, there is loss of or impaired vision. There can also be speech issues, and the most common with most of us is one side of our body is paralyzed.

Let's take a break for a second. As I was editing and reviewing this section, it occurred to me that you are already reading or listening, so why am I telling you to do something you are already doing? Instead, I will suggest that you *keep* reading because there are things I did not know and did not find out about until days, weeks, or months after I was already in rehabilitation.

There is an extraordinary amount of information and resources that I could talk about concerning everything about a stroke, but you've already had the stroke, and you know what a stroke is. My focus is on the recovery process and the things you will have to go through during recovery. You don't really need to worry about or focus on what a stroke is because you are now an expert at having a stroke, and your health care professionals will provide you with ample education. You do need to be aware of life choices and prevention. Learning more about what a stroke is can help in stroke prevention but may not necessarily prepare you on how to recover and be successful in the rehabilitation process. You will be provided with plenty of information about things to do as you move forward that will help improve your life or lifestyle.

Attitude

I'm bringing up attitude and putting this right up front that while there are a lot of steps you will go through during recovery, the main thing to be concerned about is having a positive attitude and to stay clear of the negative. It is easy to tell someone to have a positive attitude, but changing our attitude can be difficult, which is why it is so critically important to make the change right away. If you feel sorry for yourself, you will need to move past it, move forward, and attack the new challenge you have been given and win the fight.

You may not realize it or believe it, but you have been blessed. You are blessed because you are a *Stroke-Surviving Death Dodger.* If you do not believe in God, you're still blessed. Like it or not, accept it or not, you are in the next chapter of your life, and you have been handed a new puzzle piece to add to your life puzzle, and what you do with it is up to you.

Your attitude is going to make the difference in whether you have a successful recovery. I will often mention **little things**, emphasizing it's the **little things** that will make a difference in recovery and your perspective and attitude. I've known stroke victims and seen a significant difference in how attitude had a positive or negative impact on their progress.

I've done my best to keep sections in the book short and to the point and not provide you with too much information. My hope is to provide informational guidance that will help you navigate through your recovery and rehabilitation, hopefully inspiring you to look for the positives and **the little things that develop into big things and successes.** What I share with you is based on my experience and the shared experiences of other stroke survivors I've met.

THE FIRST SEVEN DAYS

The Stroke and a Minute with God

People experience a stroke at different times and under many different circumstances. My experience was on a late Monday evening in March 2022. I was in the bathroom finishing up, dried my hands, turned around toward the sink, and felt my left leg buckle. At first, I wasn't aware something was going on other than thinking, *That's odd, my left leg kind of gave way*. Then, surprise! I threw both my hands up on the bathroom sink, and it was then that I noticed that my left arm was giving way a little. Initially, I did not experience lightheadedness or anything like that. I tried my left leg again, but it was not cooperating.

I opened the bathroom door and was able to grab the doorframe to help keep my balance. The bathroom door is situated right next to a small bedroom that I use for my office With a hold on the doorframe, I made a couple of hops toward the office, grabbed onto the door handle of the office door then made a couple more hops, covering the distance— maybe three or four feet—to my desk. All this time, I still wasn't sure what was going on, but one thing was for sure, I was feeling *funny*. I made it to my desk chair and plopped down. My left arm felt heavy and was hanging down. Something was happening in my head, and I experienced a feeling of lightheadedness or the sensation of nearly passing out.

It was at this point I knew something was going on, and okay, I know, the first clue should have been a minute ago when my leg gave out. I started doing things simultaneously. I started telling myself, *stay awake, stay awake.* I reached for my cell phone on the desk but knocked it off, and it fell to the floor. I leaned over trying to grab the phone with my right hand while still focusing on staying awake. This is when reality set in and when the conversation with God started.

I felt funny or weird or whatever we want to call it. I knew something was happening, or maybe I was dying, I didn't know. *"Not now God, not now."* I knew I did not want to die. Of course, none of us wants to die. Meanwhile, I'm experiencing a rush of conflicting thoughts. I was still trying to reach the phone when an unexpected visitor appeared. Our nine-month-old gray, blue-eyed Boston terrier named Izzie started licking my right hand. People say dogs instinctively know when something is wrong, and I believe that was the case with Izzie.

The puppy kept licking my hand, which oddly helped keep my focus on grabbing the phone. My conversation with God continued as I kept trying to get the phone. *"Not now, I'm not ready,"* and I know, I know, saying I'm not ready may sound like a normal reaction or somewhat selfish when you think you might die. It's funny what people say about what goes through their minds during a near-death experience. The sudden act of someone running into a burning building, someone doing something outrageous—an act of courage, a soldier saving their buddy, or other acts ignoring their own safety or life. The sudden state of mind that switches from the natural self-preservation mode to concern and safety of others may be unexplainable, or maybe it is explainable, maybe it's love or something else. In any case, I wasn't running into a burning building, but the

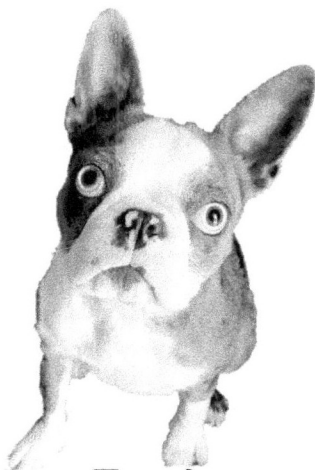

Izzie

thoughts that started to run through my head were about my family and not about myself.

I was thinking about my family and how my death would impact my wife Debbie, my kids, and our two grandsons. Debbie and I had been married 46 years, we have three kids and consider our daughter-in-law our kid too—so four kids total. Plus, since the stroke, one of our daughters got married, which brought us a son-in-law—a fifth kid—and a granddaughter.

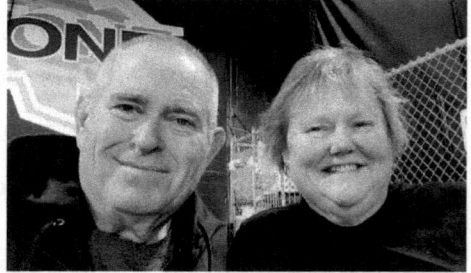

I have a very personal relationship with my grandkids, and I felt like they needed me in their lives, or at least, that is what us grandparents like to think. We lived in the same apartment complex where our son and daughter-in-law lived with their nine- and five-year-old sons. Our living there was on purpose. However, it's not an *Everyone Loves Raymond*-type of arrangement. We moved in there nine years earlier when the first grandson was born so that we could be available for babysitting. We've helped with both boys since they were born, and I even started a children's book series about our time and adventures together, AdventureswithPopPop.com. (How about that for some self-promotion!)

Back to my minute with God. My concern was how this would impact my family, and it was weird how quickly my thoughts switched from what's happening to me to what would happen to them. *"Please God."*

After about a minute, I finally was able to get hold of the phone. Okay a double "Duh" moment about trying to get my phone. I guess I could have yelled out for Debbie, but it did not occur to me. I was too focused on the phone, talking with God, and Izzie licking my hand. Debbie had already been in bed a couple of hours. I called her on her cell phone and heard her phone's distinctive ringtone. She had this funny ringtone that was a quack quack quack followed by the person's name. I heard the quacking, then "Papa Daddy," which was the name on her phone for me. She answered the phone asking what was wrong. She seemed to instinctively know something was wrong.

She asked, "What's wrong, baby?" and my reply was, "Mommy, I need help."

The way I said mommy scared her and was not very clear. She knew right away something was wrong when the way I said the word "mommy" sounded more like "mummy," like from a horror movie. I heard the bedroom door open within seconds. She asked again what's wrong and then she stopped midsentence when she saw me slumped back in the chair. A few seconds later, I heard her talking to a 911 operator.

A minute or two later, I heard the voices of the ambulance crew. I'll stop right here to compliment and praise the Creve Coeur, Missouri, fire department because, in my mind, they literally got there within two minutes. I checked later and their actual response time was four minutes, which is just as amazing. I cannot say enough about them because, although I was a little out of it—okay, a *lot* out of it—I was still conscious, or maybe it was semiconscious, answering questions and aware of what was going on. I could hear my wife talking to one of them the whole time, and the other one was talking to me. Suddenly, it felt like four of them were lifting me up and placing me on the stretcher. I say it would take at least four of them because at the time I was 270 pounds. They rolled me outside toward the ambulance.

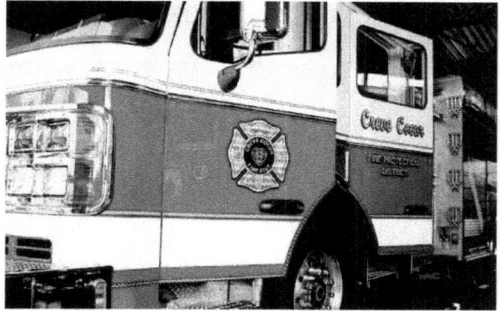

A humorous side note about what else happened. The puppy Izzie followed us out and tried to jump up into the ambulance. Debbie had already called the kids. Tanya, our daughter-in-law, was already outside and grabbed Izzie.

The ER

I heard the ambulance doors close, felt the motion of the ambulance moving, and heard the siren. They were taking me to Mercy Hospital, which was about a five-minute drive. I was very fortunate where we lived to be so close to the fire department and the hospital. One thing I was certain of was that Debbie wasn't going to lose sight of me and was probably on the bumper of the ambulance all the way to the hospital.

I remember the ambulance coming to a stop and backing up and me being taken out of the ambulance and into the ER. At this point, I don t remember much, although I did notice the brisk March night air when they rolled me into the ER. Debbie's version of the story is she was following me into the ER, and the nurses offered her a wheelchair because they could see that she was worried and stressed. Sometime later, the doctor confirmed I'd had a hemorrhagic stroke, explained everything, and reassured Debbie that I was doing good.

This is where I remember upon hearing Debbie's voice, I yelled out "Mummy" in that zombie voice. Not only did my slurred "mummy" scare her, this was also the first time she had seen me since I got to the ER. I was in the hospital bed, my legs and arms had IVs sticking into them, and I was staring up at the ceiling, zoned out. It kind of terrified her, but the doctor reassured her I was doing good.

On to the ICU

After the ER, the next stop was the ICU (Intensive Care Unit). My memory of this time is a little vague. I remember waking up. I think a nurse was telling me what was going on with me. Debbie was there, too, but not allowed to stay overnight. Depending on the situation and how severe your stroke is, you are about to enter an adjustment period, which you may not even realize at this point. I had paralysis on my left side. Weeks later when I was in outpatient therapy, I heard of some stroke victims getting out of the ICU within a day, so it all depends on your individual case. I was in the ICU for a week.

One of the goals in ICU is stabilizing and controlling things like diabetes, high blood pressure, and high cholesterol, among other things. I already had diabetes, high blood pressure, and high cholesterol. I was also overweight, and the doctors explained that these conditions were the contributing factors to the stroke. While these conditions are factors that contribute to a stroke, it's important to be clear that not everyone who has a stroke has these conditions. People of all shapes, sizes, races, ethnicities, and varying health conditions have strokes.

Day Two and Moving Forward

One of the things I noticed was the number of medications they were giving me. Instead of metformin for diabetes, they were giving me insulin shots and checking my blood sugar multiple times a day. They were also giving me blood thinners, high blood pressure, and cholesterol meds. I'm talking about a bunch of medications, which was something new.

After you've been stabilized in the ER and on to ICU, life as you knew it is in a process of continual change, and a lot of little things will be happening. You may be saying to yourself, *I know all this already. I had a stroke.* Agreed. However, family and caretakers may not know all of this, and it's important for them to understand and be aware of everything that's happening with you.

So Many Adjustments

So many adjustments are happening and will continue to happen, I'm sure I will not cover all of them. I would think that the biggest adjustment is the emotional one, learning how to cope, manage, and handle the challenge that has been given to you. There are a lot of other adjustments.

Bathroom and a Transfer/Slide Board

One adjustment, although it may not initially seem like a big one, is the bathroom. For some of us, it's not a big deal with a nurse, medical tech, or someone helping you. I know there are some people who are very modest, and it might be bothersome, but

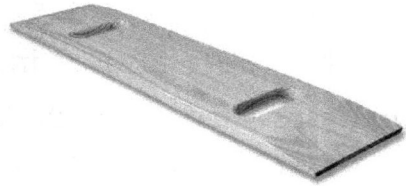

TRANSFER / SLIDE BOARD

privacy and modesty can no longer be a concern and is something to accept and get used to, especially considering if you have lost the use of one of your hands and legs. The use of a urinal will become normal, and for bowel movements, a bedpan and transition to a slide board will be used to move/slide from the wheelchair to the toilet seat. Depending on the extent of the paralysis, you may likely continue to need help with the bathroom once you get home. Remember, while it's a natural reaction to want to do things yourself or help yourself, you must remember that you need help and may continue to need help.

Dehydration

I was drinking water all the time and, as a result, was having to urinate on average every two hours, and this adjustment comes with having help with these frequent bathroom breaks.

Paralysis

Usually on the left side, the left arm and leg are paralyzed to the point where you have no control, you cannot move them, have no touch sensation, cannot feel anything, and cannot move your shoulder, all of which is a big adjustment.

The Call Button

Due to limited mobility, you need to have awareness of where the call button is for when you need help. This is both in the ICU and when you go to the rehab hospital, so you just need to create an awareness of your surroundings.

Personal Perspectives

Some patients may have a different perspective on what their disabilities may be. For many, it is paralysis, but there may also be vision loss, the inability to speak, or speaking with a slur. There are also bowel issues. There are a lot of other issues that stroke patients can experience, and each one of us handles and manages them in different ways.

Speech

Some stroke victims have severe speech issues while others do not. There may also be cognitive issues with how you function. Simple things like using a phone, a remote, or a computer that seemed simple before may now be difficult. Everyone has different effects and different levels of severity.

Vision

I was fortunate; every time the doctors visited me in the ICU and also in the rehab hospital, they always asked me how my vision was and if I could see okay. To be honest, at the time, I thought my vision was fine. After a couple of weeks, I noticed that glare was bothering me, things like a bright room light, sunlight, etc. The reality was that there were minor vision issues but not major ones. Months later, I noticed my left eye had some minor issues.

Chewing Problems

Chewing is a common problem. Initially, I could not feel the left side of my face and could not tell if there was food in the left side of my mouth. Drinking with a straw became the norm. Trying to drink out of a cup, bottle, or can would not work. Over time, the chewing issue seemed to get back to normal. Taking meds can be another problem. It was strongly suggested—and I will tell you to follow it—to take one pill at a time. A lot of people try to take two or three pills and end up choking.

Pillows

You will notice your first night and in the weeks to come, including when you go home, that they will likely put pillows underneath your legs for elevation and also under your shoulder or arm. The reason for propping the arm and shoulder is they also need to be elevated and for their tendency to hang or fall off the bed, and the pillow helps prevent that and provides stability.

The Gait Belt

Your new best friend is your **gait belt**. Among many adjustments is the gait belt. This belt is around your waist anytime you move, and it's used because you are a fall hazard. Plus, you're also not able to move on your own, so anytime you move, someone will be

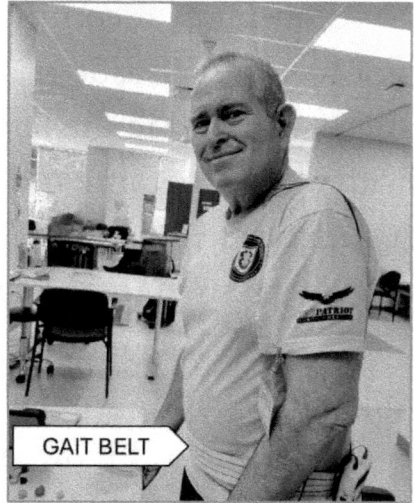

with you. This is something that continued from ICU on to the rehab hospital and when I went home.

Crossed Wires

The emotions are one part of the wires being crossed. It's amazing how everything—your muscles, your nerves, your brain—all interact. You may feel your hand is sitting by your side when it's actually on your chest or hanging off the bed.

Positive Attitude

I already mentioned attitude is everything. Your life has changed dramatically. The most important thing you can do is maintain a positive attitude and outlook. Do not dwell on what happened. Focus on the future with a positive attitude, and do not even give depression a chance to take a hold of you. Keep focused and plan for the future.

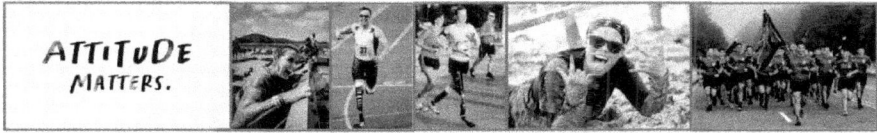

POSITIVE ATTITUDE

Winding Down ICU

Wow! Everything I've mentioned up to this point happened in just one week. The adjustments and learning to manage and navigate your new reality have happened in one week? Hopefully your stay in the ICU will be short; for me, it was a week.

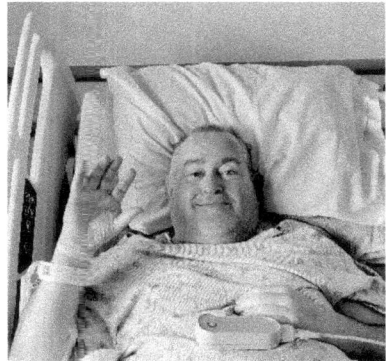

The doctors visited every day and explained everything about the stroke and the treatment plan while in the ICU. They were focusing on stabilizing me—getting the diabetes, high blood pressure, and high cholesterol under control—and preparing me for the rehab process.

The doctors had conversations with me and Debbie about sending me to the Mercy Rehabilitation

Hospital down the road in Chesterfield, Missouri. A nurse from the rehab hospital visited and gave us a briefing. If it didn't already occur to you, one thing will quickly become very clear: You are not going home, and you will need rehab. To clarify, some people do go home, but those are the less severe cases. When I was in outpatient therapy, I met quite a few people who never went to a rehab hospital. They went straight from the ICU to home but had to attend outpatient therapy. Again, this was because of the lesser severity of the stroke and the specific needs of the patient.

You Are Not the Only Victim

I mention this here because this is very important and something that may not occur to you until later. I had an epiphany of sorts one night after I'd been in the rehab hospital a few days, which was about ten days after the stroke. I was on the phone with Debbie, and she mentioned something, and it suddenly occurred to me what the stroke had done to her and my family, and the emotional toll it had taken on all of them. It was emotionally overwhelming when I realized that I was not the only victim in this situation. Of course, I was the one who had had the stroke, but it scared Debbie to death plus incurred lots of other emotions.

It affected my kids and grandkids, and that knowledge or realization didn't hit me until that night.

My point about bringing this up is while having a stroke or injury may be devasting to the individual, it is also devastating to the family. It can be easy to ignore or not even notice how they are affected. I noticed during the months I was going to outpatient therapy that there were a few patients who treated their spouses or caretakers terribly, demeaning them and being hateful toward them. It was also noticeable that some spouses were exhausted, emotionally drained, and having trouble dealing with their situation.

The first few days after a stroke is only the beginning. Family and friends are concerned and can be emotionally impacted. You may have dodged death and felt like you could have died, but we need to remember that family can also be traumatized by the thought that they could have lost you.

The Emotions Are Coming

The flood of emotions experienced after a stroke reminds me of a line from a Robin Williams stand-up performance: "The emotions are coming!" Aside from all the other issues, emotions can be bothersome and, sometimes, a major obstacle. Almost all stroke victims experience a big change in emotions and what some of us call our *filters*. By filters, I mean doing things you didn't previously do, like verbal outbursts or getting upset about something. We may very easily get sad, mad, cry, or experience many other variations in the emotional spectrum. I'm jumping ahead to tell you about how during the first few months I was home, I found that I was jumpy, getting nervous over nothing, and sometimes I would react angrily and not at anything in particular. These were reactions with no real explanation, which took some adjusting for family members... I'm fibbing here. It's not *some* adjusting, it takes *a lot* of adjusting.

One day we were watching a movie. I've never cried at movies before, but there we were watching *Father Stu*, a Mark Wahlberg movie, 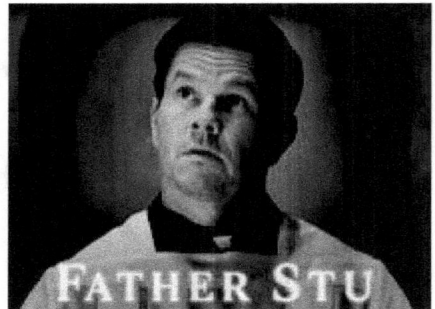 and Debbie looked over at me and asked, "Are you crying?" I said, "I guess so." Of all the movies to be emotional about, it was a Mark Wahlberg movie. I really do like Wahlberg movies, so no disrespect to Wahlberg, but the fact it was a Mark Wahlberg movie makes us laugh now at that memory.

Another thing about the emotions is that some stroke victims don't realize that their filters have been altered. It can be difficult to get a stroke victim to acknowledge it. Once I became a little self-aware, my solution to my changes was to joke about it using the line, "I got an excuse," and that lightened the mood and others' reactions. Another problem is that initially some family members or caretakers do not know or understand that it's a side effect and not on purpose or to be taken personally. The changes with emotions may not be permanent. I've noticed that over time, I have adjusted and developed—or redeveloped—patience...or that's what I tell myself. Patience is important. I've been told that I'm still a little jumpy.

REHAB HOSPITAL: THE NEXT THREE WEEKS

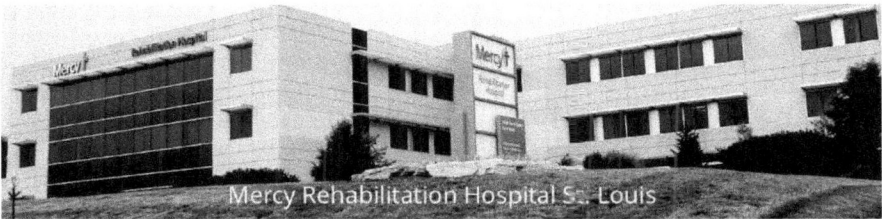
Mercy Rehabilitation Hospital St. Louis

At this point, it's only been a week, so remember, everything mentioned up to now, the adjustments and little things, are still happening. You may ask what is a rehabilitation hospital? I will keep it short because a lot of what happens at the rehab hospital continues after you leave and go to outpatient therapy. I guess one way to explain a rehab hospital is that it is a three-week prep for a longer rehabilitation progress. The reality of a stroke is different for everyone, although rehab and recovery are similar. On rare occasions, a stroke victim is up and walking around, or back to normal, within a week or two. Most of us have the same typical effects from a stroke. The rehab starts at the rehab hospital, and it's generally two or three weeks. After that, you are sent home for in-home therapy or outpatient therapy at a facility.

After seven days in the ICU, I was cleared to be transferred to the rehab hospital. This happened on Monday evening. The rehab hospital wanted me there Monday morning so they could start my rehab, but my transfer was delayed by what should have been a simple thing—a bowel movement, or in my case, the lack thereof. After the momentous bowl movement, I had an ambulance ride to the rehab hospital. They got me processed and into what would be my room for the next three weeks, room 237. The staff worked twelve-hour shifts that switched over at seven. There was a primary nurse and a medical technician (med tech).

They got me all set up and later after dinner, they helped me into a hospital gown for the night. Next morning, they came in and woke me up around 5:30, giving me a schedule for the day that showed meal and therapy session times. I felt like wow, they're not wasting any time.

The nurse did the morning vitals check, gave me meds, and the med tech got me dressed, and then I went for my second flying lesson in the rehab hospital. I forgot to mention when I got there the night before, they introduced me to this contraption called a Hoyer lift; another name for it is a burrito bag. They have this canvas shell you sit in that is hooked up to a ceiling hoist that is used to hoist you out of the wheelchair and into the bed or out of the bed and into the chair. I already started entertaining the staff because as soon as they hoisted me out of bed, I yelled "Weeeeeeeee," like that little piggy in the old Geico insurance television commercials.

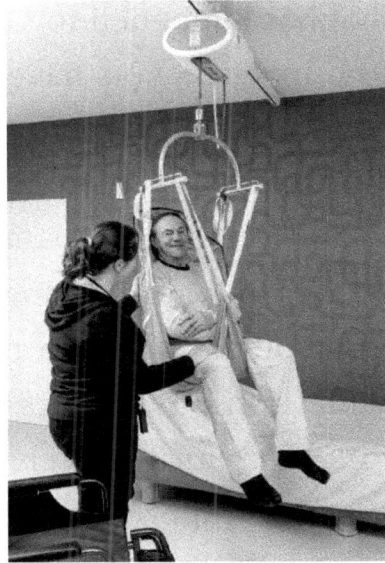

The physical therapist doctor, Dr. Thorley, stopped in to see me early. The visit lasted about ten minutes and was thorough. He explained who he was and what his role was and provided me with one of the best explanations I've heard about a stroke. The view from my room's window looked out on Interstate 64, and he used this analogy: "Imagine for a second that a bomb just blew up out there on the highway. That is what has happened to your brain—a bomb exploded. Now imagine you have construction crews that are repairing that highway out there. You have the same thing happening to your brain and body."

Dr. Thorley's explanation made sense. Our bodies are amazing at repairing themselves, and so basically your body is going to rebuild itself—the wiring, the connections, the nerves—all these things are going to work to repair themselves. This is one of the reasons you may experience nerve pain even months later because the body is working to repair itself. When I asked about the timeline, he straightforwardly told me there is no real timeline because everyone is different. It could be a month, it could be three months, six months, a year, or longer. Everyone's progress is different. His explanation, although not a definitive answer, was encouraging.

By the time 7 a.m. came around, the med tech wheeled me out of my room and headed downstairs to the cafeteria for breakfast. One of the adjustments you're going to make is how you spend your day. During my time at the rehab hospital, I made the comment that I felt like I was back in the Army because I was put on a schedule, up at 5:30, with three meals a day. Your day is planned out for you just like in the military or basic training. You're told where to go, how to get there, when to be there, and the same thing is pretty much the same with the rehab hospital. There was a schedule for meals and therapy sessions in between meals throughout the day.

Another adjustment was the diet. If you are diabetic, they'll put you on a diabetic diet, which continued from what I was on in the ICU. Every night I turned in a menu for the next day. I thought the options were not that bad, but then again, I'm an ex-army guy, so I'm used to cafeteria-type food.

In the cafeteria, you'll get parked at a table and there's cafeteria staff and a nurse supervisor. The nurse is there for a lot of reasons, one being you are considered a choking

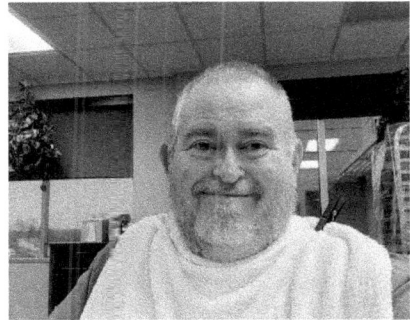

BIG BOY BIB AND SCRUFFY BEARD

hazard. It may not have affected you that way, but initially they will keep an eye on you. You may have a name tag on you that says, "choking hazard," and they'll put a Big Boy Bib on you in case you drool or make a mess.

I did not have problems with chewing or swallowing (that's what I thought), but some stroke victims do have those issues, which is why they put the bib on you and why they keep an eye on you. In hindsight, I did have some problems with swallowing because when taking meds, I would sometimes choke on them. So, yes, even if you don't think you have a problem, you probably do.

Changing Your Eating Habits

Some stroke victims may have developed bad eating habits like I had, or your upbringing contributed to developing the habit of eating large portions, drinking a lot of soda, snacking, and just overindulging. In hindsight, I will admit I was guilty of that. If there was a positive that came from this stroke, it was that during the three to four weeks in the hospital and rehab hospital, I made a complete change in my eating habits. Although it was regulated, it was beneficial to me and changed everything about my food and drink intake and eliminated cravings. I quit soda, converted to small portions, and just made an overall change to my diet that continued after I went home. During the combined four weeks in the hospitals, I lost around 30 pounds, and within the first two months after going home, I lost another 40 pounds for a total weight loss of 70 pounds.

Starting Rehabilitation Therapy

Let's continue my story about my first morning. While I was sitting there eating breakfast, a woman walked over to my table and sat down. Her name was Lynn, and she introduced herself as a speech therapist and that she was going to sit with me during breakfast so she could observe how I eat. There it was—therapy had already started during breakfast.

When I finished breakfast, Lynn rolled me up to the second floor to her office where we spent about an hour. Lynn reviewed a lot with me, explaining what speech therapy was all about. One misconception about speech therapy is that it's only about talking and using our voice. There is more to it involving areas related to cognitive issues, reading ability, and even how you chew and swallow.

The Three Therapies

Therapy is broken down into three areas or categories: speech therapy, occupational therapy, and physical therapy. Each of the three sessions are usually an hour each, totaling three hours a day. I've kept this part a bit short because the therapy continues after the rehab hospital at outpatient therapy, so I'll go into more detail later.

Speech Therapy (ST)

Speech therapy may sound like it's just about speech, but it's more than that. Speech therapy sessions are usually an hour a day and cover working on audio skills, vocal exercises, reading, calculating, and other cognitive skill exercises called executive functioning. Spending an hour in speech therapy can be tiring, even more so than the physical therapy at times.

Occupational Therapy (OT)

OT is focused on working with you on your personal functions and daily tasks, such as how to dress yourself, move from a chair to a bed, and getting on and off the toilet. You'll likely be introduced to an arm sling and continue to use a sling for months (keep in mind, my severity may have been worse than yours).

Physical Therapy (PT)

PT is focused on your physical abilities, muscle development, and getting you to stand up and work on taking steps. The therapist may start with a harness to hoist you up on your feet or try several other techniques to work on standing. They may also test a brace to give your foot stability; the affected foot has a tendency to curve or bend inward, and a brace retrains your foot to stay in its normal position.

Usually, the three therapies are generally an hour each day, five days a week, and split up during the day. You'll probably be very tired from all this, depending on your individual situation, strength level, and ability to concentrate. The rehab hospitals are limited by insurance, so depending on your insurance, there may be a time limit for how long you can stay. For me, it was three weeks, and from there, it's off to outpatient therapy, where the three therapies continue and are more extensive.

Super Tired and Sleep, Sleep, Sleep

The rehab sessions are tiring, and you may find opportunities during the day to take a nap. I found that I was sleeping ten to twelve hours a night. As soon as dinner was over, I was out for the night, and this continued for months, even after I went home. The doctors told me that sleep was good because your body is repairing itself while you're sleeping.

Where's My Leg and Where's My Arm?

Within a day or a few days after the stroke, one thing that I became very aware of was wondering,

"Where is my leg?" or "where is my arm?" That may sound funny, but what I discovered was I had no sensation and no awareness of where they were. If someone forgot to put the bed rail up, you could find your leg dangling off the side of the bed, or when you're sitting in a wheelchair, your arm is dangling or fell off the armrest. This is one thing you must get used to and create an awareness of where they are, so you don't injure yourself. This is coupled with what is called "heavy leg" or "heavy arm," which has something to do with **spasticity**.

An abundance of information is out there that can explain spasticity and the occurrence of heavy leg and heavy arm. One explanation I found was that after a stroke, the muscles may become limp and feel heavy. The muscles may shorten and become very tight, making them more difficult to move and stretch. This is called spasticity. These changes in muscle tone can affect joint stability and movement. Another explanation is called post-stroke edema, which is extra fluid buildup in the leg (or arm), making it feel heavy.

While you're still in the rehab hospital, it's very likely that this heavy leg and heavy arm feeling is not going to go away anytime soon. For me, it was several months down the road during outpatient therapy before I lost that heavy sensation, although it does come back on occasion. One of the many remedies you'll find to help is called **motor control retraining**, which is a long term for exercise. Motor control retraining is a way to strengthen all the areas of the brain that are necessary to perform a specific movement. With a heavy leg, the goal is to relearn how to bend the knee and hip.

Repetition, Repetition, Repetition!

The short definition mentioned on spasticity is not something you may notice immediately after a stroke. You may start to notice it at a later time when you start regaining some control over your arm and leg. The spasticity, tightening of ligaments and muscles, will become apparent to you and will also be associated with nerve pain. The joint area is a main area for spasticity, occurring in the elbow, wrist, shoulder, knee, hip, and hip flexor muscle.

Visitors and Distractions

Knowing that the rehab hospital stay is going to probably be three weeks, any visitors and distractions are very much appreciated. You'll probably be extremely tired, while at times, your mind may be speeding. However, a visitor is a nice distraction and can help with maintaining a positive attitude.

One of my most appreciated distractions was my family, including my two grandsons. I've already mentioned my two grandsons, whom I call the Grandmen. After the arrival of the first grandson, I became one of those obnoxious grandparents showing pictures of the Grandman on Facebook. A friend suggested I write a book about my adventures with them, and so I did, resulting in the "Adventures with Pop Pop" children's book series that I mentioned earlier.

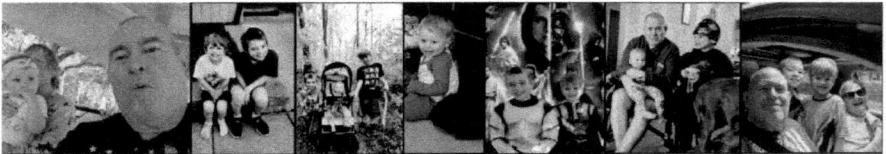

Aside from family, social media was a good distraction. I knew a lot of people within the military, writing community, and other groups of friends and family on social media, where I was active. There I found a lot of interaction and encouragement, which helped. I started to post updates on Facebook on my situation and progress, which I continued to do. The responses, comments, and prayers were encouraging and a big help. I found later that my postings on Facebook were encouraging to others, which was an unexpected plus.

I would strongly suggest that you share your experience, good or bad. You'll find it to be therapeutic and encouraging, not just for yourself, but to others as well.

Staying Busy

Aside from a good distraction, staying busy is very important, even when your ability to return to work may be limited. You may also be retired or semi-retired, like in my case. I was 66 years old when I had the stroke and had been retired from the army for over twenty years. I worked a part-time job teaching online business courses. I was fortunate to be able to continue working because it was a good distraction and kept my brain active.

I'm sure continuing to work helped me cope with my situation, as did writing and having visitors. Aside from my family, I had other people I know visit, plus I had tremendous support and interaction on Facebook.

The second morning at the rehab hospital, the doctor saw my laptop and asked what I was doing. I told him about my work and added, "I don't have an off switch." The doctor found this humorous and encouraging and noted that it was a good thing to be able to keep the mind doing work. In hindsight, working was a tremendous contribution to my recovery and provided me with this insight: *Keep your brain busy.*

I would add at this point that while you may not actually be able to do physical work, keeping your mind busy—finding things to do like writing, reading, or listening to audiobooks like you are doing right now—is helpful for your recovery.

Speech-to-Text Technology

I quickly adapted to using my right hand on the computer keyboard and learned how to use speech-to-text technology. As time passed, I found that speech-to-text technology was a valuable tool because it drew my attention to what I was saying. I found that I was slurring speech, mispronouncing words, and had problems articulating my words, simply not making sense at times. The speech-to-text application was a very useful tool that helped me improve my verbalization.

Your New Ride

I'm making the assumption you are wheelchair-bound, and by the time of your third (or last) week at the rehab hospital, you should receive your new wheelchair. One thing I learned a little later about wheelchairs is that the height is adjustable, which could make a difference in your ability to get out of the chair or stand up. Wheelchairs may also need a tune-up, and the medical supply company that provided it will service the chair. They'll even make house calls and see you at the outpatient therapy facility.

Listen to Your Spouse/Partner
My Wife Was Angry

Debbie had been upset with me about wanting my laptop at the ICU, but that was not the real reason she was upset. For years, Debbie had fussed at me about my high blood pressure. If you're unfamiliar with the term, *fuss* is another word for getting upset, among other things. My primary doctor had diagnosed me with diabetes and high blood pressure six years prior in 2016. The doctor had prescribed medication for diabetes; however, he had not prescribed medication for high blood pressure, which was a repeated question asked by the ICU and rehab doctors as well as my new primary doctor.

Debbie was angry and upset with me, rightfully so, because I hadn't listened to her suggestions about getting treated for high blood pressure and working on a healthier diet or lifestyle, plus she was also angry with my doctor for not treating me for the high blood pressure. On a side note, I had known better about my health given my years as a karate guy, runner, and being in the army, and yet, even though I knew better, I still ignored it. There's always hindsight. So, if you happen to be, or know someone, who is older, maybe retired from the military, and find yourself gaining weight and not being as active as you used to be, you (or they) really need to stop what you're doing and fix it.

My point is to listen to your spouse and family when they fuss about your health and making changes, and while they may be angry with you, it's because they love and care about you. Remember to listen to that voice in your head suggesting you go for a run or go to the gym, and don't listen to the lazy voice telling you to go back to sleep or that it's too cold or too hot.

I Quit

I think it's important to talk about "I Quit" here. Our attitudes can have a significant impact on our life, even more of a positive or negative impact than any physical limitation. A positive attitude is critical for positive results. I didn't quit, but I know of someone who did. Quitting and giving up is something you cannot do.

I am a retired army guy and spent most of my career in Special Forces (Green Berets). I am a member of our local Special Forces association chapter, and we have a lot of supporters who help with fundraising events and other activities—people like Mary Jo, who gave me permission to share her story.

On my third day at the rehabilitation hospital in the therapy gym, I saw a woman walking out at the far end who was the spitting image of Mary Jo. Later that evening, I got on Facebook and messaged her, asking if she was at the rehab hospital. Her answer was yes; her sister Donna had had a stroke, and she had been visiting her.

I bring this up, not only because of what a small world it is, but also as an example of how our attitude can be more debilitating than the physical limitations that a stroke or injury can inflict on us.

A few days later, Mary Jo was in the cafeteria at lunchtime with her sister. We chatted, and Mary Jo expressed concern for Donna because she was not doing well emotionally, was depressed, and wanted to go home. I saw Donna and Mary Jo almost daily in the cafeteria. Donna was eating in the cafeteria, doing her exercises, and participating in activities, but her heart wasn't in it. Donna arranged to move into a nursing home and quit all the therapy and rehab activities she had been instructed to do and stopped participating in her own recovery and rehabilitation. During the 18 months after her stroke, Donna lacked a positive and hopeful attitude, she lost 70 pounds, and to put it simply, she gave up.

Donna passed away 18 months after the stroke. Our point for sharing this is to emphasize how important it is to cultivate, encourage, and maintain a positive attitude. During my 10 months in outpatient therapy, I met and interacted with dozens who all agreed that attitude is by far our most important tool in recovery and moving forward.

Don't let depression get ahold of you.
Don't quit!

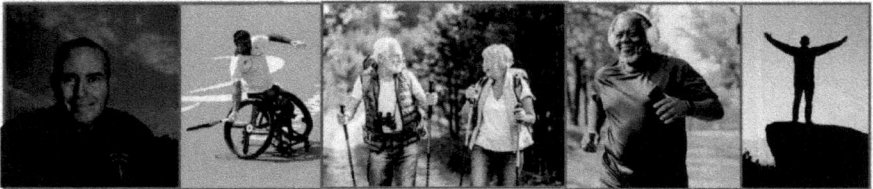

Don't Stop, Don't Give Up, Don't Quit

DISCHARGE FROM THE REHAB HOSPITAL

Heading Home

Four weeks since the stroke, a lot has happened and a lot more was in store. I was discharged from the hospital on a Tuesday morning, which was exciting and also the first time I'd been outside and gotten some fresh air. Going home was nice for many reasons, especially for the grandkids who were excited to see me home. They made me "Welcome Home" posters.

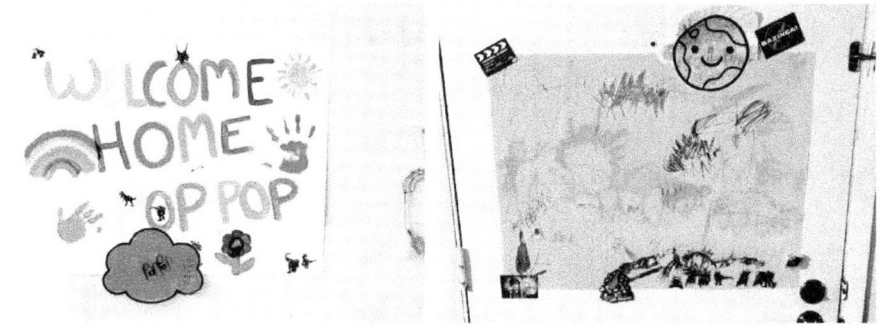

The staff at the rehab hospital had talked with Debbie to arrange for a hospital bed and bedside commode to be delivered to the apartment, marking another adjustment. Chances are that when you were in the ICU and the rehab hospital, you were sleeping slightly elevated and will probably continue to do this for a while. Insurance usually pays for these items.

We also ordered a bench for the bathtub and portable ramps for the wheelchair to use on the front door and breezeway steps. The medications I was on in the hospital continued for the time being, except the insulin shots were changed to metformin.

Items You May Need When You Go Home
- Gait belt
- Transfer board
- Hospital bed
- Bedside commode
- Commode liners
- Bathtub bench
- Reacher/grabber tool
- Portable ramp
- Grab bars
- Blood pressure monitor (arm type, not wrist)
- Blood glucose test kit

- Pill box
- And 20 other things you'll think of

A Few Other Things Before Outpatient Therapy

You may experience these other things during this time of transition and should be aware of them. When you first go home, a lot of things will happen. Although you'll be glad you're home, there are adjustments. Depending on your home, you may find that the wheelchair will not fit through the bathroom door. Waaaaa.

A few months later, we ordered grab bars for the shower and had them installed. The apartment we lived in was not handicap accessible. Since we were comfortable where we were, we did not plan on moving. In hindsight, I wish we had made the apartment more accessible earlier in my recovery. I did learn from the guy who installed the grab bars that the Veterans Administration will provide and install grab bars and ramps at no cost to veterans. It does not take very long to get that accomplished.

The Floor Feels Different

"The floor feels different," I realized, and it would impact my recovery. When I left the rehab hospital, I was still in a wheelchair, and the few steps I did take in physical therapy were on a hard surface—a tile floor. Once home, it would be a few weeks before I was able to venture out of the wheelchair. As the days passed in physical therapy, I was walking on a hard surface. But our apartment had carpeted floors, and my first attempt at home to take a few steps felt really weird. It turns out that the slightest little thing disrupts your balance and ability to navigate, even something like carpet versus hard flooring. It took several weeks and much effort to adjust to different floor surfaces. This also happens outside with slight inclines.

Fatigue Factor

Tiredness is a normal side effect. Post-stroke fatigue (PSF) is a common feeling of exhaustion or tiredness that can occur at any point during the recovery process after a stroke. It's different from typical tiredness because it's not always related to recent activity and doesn't usually improve with rest. The doctors told me that it's normal, similar to what they told me about needing more hours of sleep.

Nerve Pain

Let's not forget about nerve pain. You may initially experience nerve pain right after the stroke or not until sometime later. Nerve pain can be described as shooting, stabbing, burning, prickling, electric shock, or pins and needles.

Within the first few months after the stroke, a lot of neurological activity occurs. Aside from nerves working overtime to try to adjust and heal, simple things like a friendly tap on the arm or leg may result in a loud "Owie." Or if someone was helping put a sock on or off and dropped your foot...well, if you've ever seen the classic Christmas movie *A Christmas Story* and remember the scene when the dad has the meltdown in the basement, letting out an assortment of undistinguishable profanities, that's what it can feel like. The resulting nerve pain can be indescribable except by the use of a movie scene analogy.

A drop of the foot isn't the only cause. Because of your lack of awareness of your limbs, your wheelchair could begin moving forward and you forget to pick your foot up, resulting in it getting pulled under the chair, resulting in more profanity-laden owies. The arm and hand have similar nerve pain issues, especially in OT when working on new stretches and movements that result in smiling grimaces that I'll mention in a later section.

Many or most of the exercises in OT deal with improving dexterity and range of motion. These exercises generate nerve pain from the stretching or bending of the ligaments and muscles. Even the smallest movement in the fingers can generate nerve pain. Often I would joke about the nerve pain by thinking, "at least I am feeling something." My therapist would ask me about my pain, and instead of using the number scale of one to ten, I would say, "Tolerable," which became the term I used often and shared with other patients. Over time, the more stretching and exercising you do with your arm, hand, and leg, the less nerve pain you will experience.

Spasms

Night spasms are another source of nerve pain. During my time conversing with other patients at outpatient therapy, the different patients had a wide spectrum of experiences with nerve pain. Your neurologist will likely prescribe medication. I was initially prescribed gabapentin and later switched to baclofen, two of the most common medications prescribed for spasms. As time passed and nerve repair and exercising continued, my experience was that the nerve pain subsided, although I experienced occasional night spasms, but oddly no severe nerve pain, just muscle contractions.

Spasticity

Initially after a stroke, you likely will not notice spasticity, mainly because of the limpness of the arm and leg, although a few weeks post-stroke, you'll start to experience it. One of many definitions for **spasticity** is that it's a condition in which muscles stiffen or tighten, preventing normal fluid movement. After a stroke, muscles may become stiff, tighten up, and resist stretching. Spasticity relates to muscle tone. Tone is the natural tension, or contraction, in a muscle that resists stretching.

During a session with my trainer, who I started to use after discharge from outpatient therapy, the idea of "tough" versus "tender" hit me. It's my own explanation about how spasticity affects us. Spasticity tightens our ligaments, making them **tough**, whereas normal ligaments are **tender**, allowing them to move and be flexible.

A month after the stroke, I started outpatient therapy. A persistent issue was heavy arm and leg, compounded within a few weeks with spasticity effects. One area affected in particular was the left hip flexor muscle, which generated severe nerve pain. Stretching exercises helped. The elbow was another area that was very resistant to straightening out. During occupational therapy sessions, exercises to straighten the elbow were difficult and caused nerve pain, which, silly me, I always considered a good thing because at least I was experiencing some sort of sensation.

Unfortunately, spasticity may always be an issue. As I experienced a few months after leaving outpatient therapy, it became more severe, causing a setback due to what I humorously would say was the leg and arm talking to each other. That left hip flexor would talk to the upper left body, simultaneously constricting both body parts and causing a struggle to maintain balance. This simultaneous movement resulted in me taking one step at a time instead of continuous stepping. Trial and error will eventually help with overcoming this type of setback. It's important to find the right exercises, tools, and other remedies to help your situation.

Toddler Effect and Recovery

I added this part here when I was finishing up the book. I was watching my almost one-year-old granddaughter doing her best to walk when it hit me.

My daughter reminded me that they told us at the rehab hospital how stroke victims are like toddlers as we're trying to learn how to walk all over again. It's cute and can be a little humorous watching a toddler learning to walk, learning to control their arms and legs as they bounce around, struggling to gain their balance. That is very similar to what stroke victims experience and is a good analogy explaining the issue with the arm and leg.

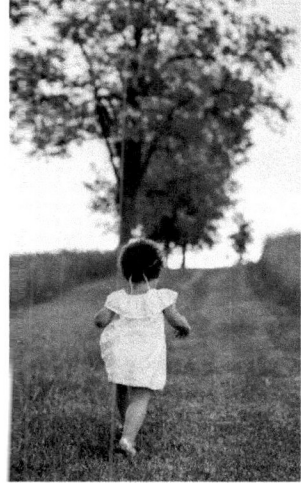

OUTPATIENT THERAPY: THE FIFTH WEEK

Outpatient therapy began the fifth week after the stroke. Debbie made sure to get me registered for outpatient therapy at SSM Health Day Institute in Chesterfield, Missouri.

SSM Health Day Institute

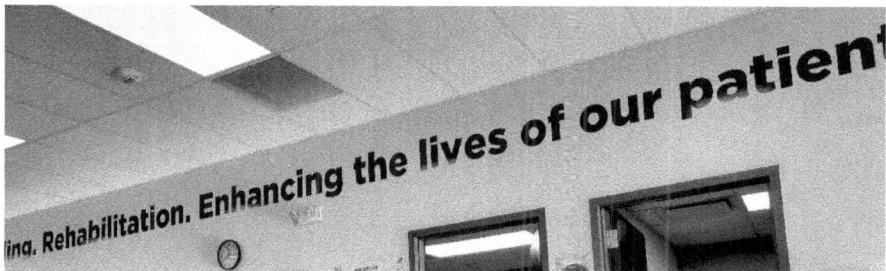

The outpatient therapy at the Day Institute and other rehabilitation facilities provides specialized, multidisciplinary care, or comprehensive care. SSM Health Day Institute specializes in a "rehabilitation program designed for individuals recovering from a traumatic injury or illness who no longer require 24-hour nursing or acute rehabilitative care" (https://www.ssmphysicaltherapy.com/services/day-institute).

Family Meeting and Training

I bring this up here because you and your family will likely have a lot of questions when starting outpatient therapy. Within a few weeks after starting outpatient therapy, a family meeting will be scheduled to review everything. In addition to a family meeting, family training can be scheduled to go over things like getting in and out of a car, negotiating steps at home, or to answer any other questions.

Starting Rehabilitation Therapy

First thing Wednesday morning, I was up, the family got me in the wheelchair and rolled me out to meet the transportation bus from the Day Institute, which at the time we thought was a good idea. So by 7 a.m., I was on my way. The bad news was within about two minutes on the bus, which was one of those minivans, I was getting nauseous, carsick, or whatever we want to call it. I would find out two to three weeks later that this was brought on by the metformin, the diabetic medicine I was on.

Day One at Outpatient Therapy

When you show up on day one, you will go through processing, orientation, paperwork, and an evaluation to assess where you are at in your recovery. You'll also be introduced to what therapy will be about. The Day Institute and all the rehab facilities are comprehensive therapy programs that follow similar approaches and therapy practices. Generally, they are a five-day-a-week program that provides speech, occupational, and physical therapies, plus a couple of hours of activities including lunchtime. I noticed that some patients attended only two, three, or four days, which seemed to be attributed to their individual needs and severity of their stroke and not necessarily due to insurance limitations that anyone mentioned.

Unfortunately, I had to go home early on my first day because I was sick from that van ride, and I also missed the next day. My family drove me to and from the Day Institute from that third day forward. I will say there is nothing wrong with the bus if you're not having problems with nausea. It was another positive for patients who did not have accessible transportation, so if you have the opportunity to take a bus/van, I would recommend it.

My first full day was Friday. Sessions were an hour each for speech, occupational, and physical therapy. The environment at outpatient therapy was nice and encouraging, and moving forward, I'll just call it rehab.

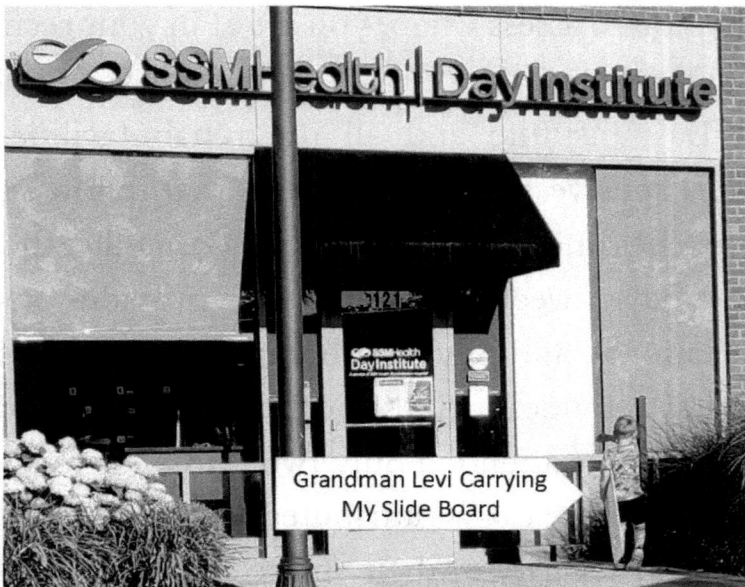

Grandman Levi Carrying My Slide Board

Everyone who worked there was enthusiastic, loved what they were doing, and were very dedicated. The therapist knew their jobs and had personalities that, I would say, were conducive to the environment they were working in. They knew how to interact with their patients, even the difficult ones. Yes, there are difficult patients.

I was impressed with the therapists who were young and had their master's or doctorate degrees in their specialty. It was nice to see younger people with such dedication to what they were doing. Okay, full disclaimer: I'm old, so I think 25 to 30 is young.

In addition to therapists, therapy aids were there to help. They loved interacting with all of us and helping as needed, like with the restroom, getting situated upon arrival, assisting with lunch, or getting a cup of coffee for the coffee drinkers. There was a running joke when a patient asked one of the therapy aides for a cup of coffee and she would ask, "What kind of coffee, regular coffee or dumb coffee?" and sometimes the answer was dumb coffee when a patient preferred decaf.

We Don't Need No Stinkin' Badges

On your first day, you will be given a badge with your name. The badge was red and has an assortment of letters that identify your status, capabilities, and limitations. The red badge is usually the first one, then as you progress, you'll earn an orange badge followed by a yellow badge. Each badge signifies your continued progress, improvement, and requirements for observation by the staff.

Manners Matter

This is another important topic that I want to point out: Manners matter. Just because we had a stroke does not mean you should be RUDE. Please and thank you. Remember when I mentioned the emotions and how wiring gets crossed? Here, too, there is a difference between speaking and saying things on purpose and saying things that you are not controlling. When it's in your control, use your manners with those helping you. Please and thank you.

Appointments Don't Stop

I encourage you to remember to never take a day off. You'll find that there's unforeseen circumstances that prevent you from going to rehab every day, like doctor's appointments, a family event, or bad weather like snow or ice. However, just because you're not physically at rehab does not mean you should not continue your training: do your homework. I use the example of runners or swimmers who, unlike most other athletes, never take a day off. They do not take a day off because even if it's raining, snowing, it's too hot or cold, they still train every day, and that's what we have to do every day. We have to always exercise and train.

The In-Between and Rest of the Day

During your days at outpatient therapy, the schedule will be spread out over an eight-hour day: six thirty-minute therapy sessions adding up to one hour a day for each type of therapy. At first, you may think that's only three hours, so what am I doing the rest of the time? You will quickly learn that the days are long and tiring. It's been a month or less since the stroke, and you're still probably sleeping ten plus hours a day, experiencing nerve pain, post-stroke fatigue, and an assortment of other things. The in-between I reference is not from the Netflix science fiction series *Stranger Things*, but a reference to what you do in between the therapy sessions.

There's a thirty-minute lunch break and discussion breakout groups, where you talk about and share experiences and tips on handling the varying situations the participants are going through. There are thirty-minute activity sessions interacting with other patients, and a personal activity book with a variety of activities designed for cognitive work. **Cognitive work** is important, and while many of us may not be aware of it at the time, in hindsight we realize, we really needed to work on our cognitive skills. You may not be a fan of board games, but that's part of the in-between activities, and it really does help with our thinking and ability to apply what is called **executive functioning**. In addition, as you gain more strength, you can spend your in-between time working on occupational therapy exercises your therapist has suggested. There is always something you can be doing.

MEET YOUR THERAPIST

On the first day of orientation, you spend some time with each of the therapists: speech, occupational, and physical. They will explain the process and do evaluations to see where you are at. While you'll likely meet your primary therapist that first day, there will be times when schedules change and you'll occasionally have different therapists. You'll get on a schedule, which will take some adjusting to get used to it. However, it will soon become routine, and you will see progress.

Speech Therapy (ST)

I have found that some people do not like speech therapy, but it is necessary, and you should absolutely not avoid it. The stroke affects everyone differently but also, in many ways, the same, and the purpose of speech therapy is not just about learning how to talk again. Some people don't have any problem with the actual physical talking part, but speech is also part of what is concerned with cognitive skills, the ability to read, do a puzzle, or some sort of word problem and other tasks. Many of the sessions are focused on executive functioning, cognitive skill building, and exercises designed to work our brains. You may be surprised to find that something you would have considered an easy task ends up being difficult.

Self-awareness of our ability can be an issue. We may feel we're processing thoughts correctly, but in fact, we are not, such as identifying five objects in a picture or comprehending the content of a paragraph. Exercises like these during sessions are part of the overall purpose of speech therapy.

One of the side effects of a stroke can be that we don't necessarily know how we've been affected. My speech was a little raspy and slightly slurred. After a few months, they sent me to a speech pathologist to get my throat checked out. There, we discovered that the stroke had affected some of my vocal cords. There was nothing seriously damaged, but there was a need to exercise those muscles, and over time, they would recover, which they did. Believe it or not, they may even have you try yodeling as a therapeutic exercise.

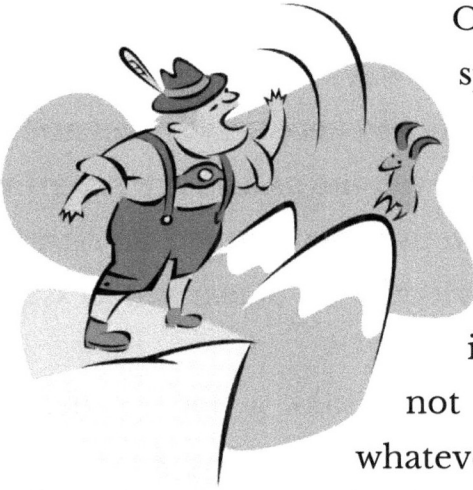

Over the months in speech therapy, I did observe some patients who were clearly experiencing cognitive and verbalization issues. This may or may not be your situation, but whatever your challenges, you will need to accept and tackle them to move forward. I was fortunate that after several months, I graduated from speech therapy, which extended my daily time an additional half hour in both occupational and physical therapy.

I'm sorry if I just scared you when I mentioned "several months," because if you weren't fully aware yet, rehab may end up being months. In my case, it lasted ten months.

Occupational Therapy (OT)

The main purpose of occupational therapy (OT) is to assist stroke victims to regain function and learn new ways to perform their daily activities, like taking a shower, grooming, dressing, and feeding yourself.

Sessions consist of activities and exercises to help with cognition, movement, vision, and occupational performance. Evaluations, activities, and tests are used to assess strengths and find ways to identify activities to help with rehabilitation and recovery. Assessment testing is administered to evaluate and gauge progress and determine the next steps for continued therapy. A goal is to help stroke victims to relearn necessary activities of daily living.

The previous paragraph said a lot to define occupational therapy. Practically speaking, all of this is blended into sessions aimed at repetitive exercises that force us to move and try, try again. Exercises include picking up a marble or another object that requires using your fingers, squeezing a ball, or grabbing small rubber objects out of a bucket and placing them on a table while also extending your arm to reach, which also serves as working on range of motion. Everything you do is intended to improve range of motion, dexterity, and your overall ability to perform individual tasks.

I started wearing a sling in the rehab hospital and continued wearing one for several more months until the therapist ordered a different type of sling for me called a **GivMohr Sling** that is *"designed to reduce shoulder subluxation and support the flaccid upper extremity in a functional position during activities in standing and ambulation"* (www.givmohrsling.com). Transitioning to this sling was a big help to me while walking and provided a more natural placement and movement of the arm.

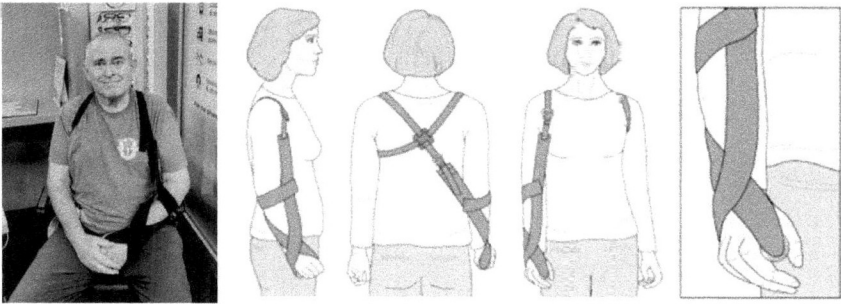

One of the first exercises they started with was moving my shoulder. At this point, it's four to five weeks after the stroke, and you're still not able to move your shoulder much, and your arm is always in a sling. You start with an exercise trying to raise and roll your shoulder in conjunction with sitting straight and squeezing your shoulder blades together. Doing this on your own will be beneficial—in fact, any exercises you can do on your own will speed up your progress, and I was eventually able to move my shoulder. A variety of exercises help with the arm, hand, and fingers. You'll probably notice that the shoulder may be one of the first major accomplishments you attain.

Monthly evaluations are used to measure your progress and are conducted for all three of the therapies. In occupational therapy, the improvements that occur from month to month are amazing. Tests to evaluate your progress measure the inches you gain, your range of motion, the number of items you can pick up in a minute, as well as other definable measurements.

One test utilizes a hand dynamometer that is used to measure grip strength.

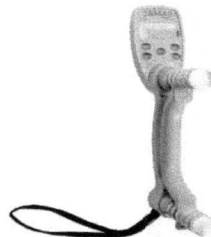

Dynamometer

An electronic pinch gauge measures pinch strength. Occupational therapy is full of activities that keep you busy and tired.

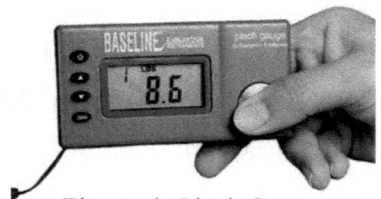

Electronic Pinch Gauge

An electrical muscle stimulator (EMS) is another tool you may be introduced to. I was introduced to this machine at the rehab hospital for my arm and continued using it in my outpatient OT sessions. I ended up being prescribed one that insurance paid for, but if insurance does not pay, the one I got cost around two hundred dollars. I used one called

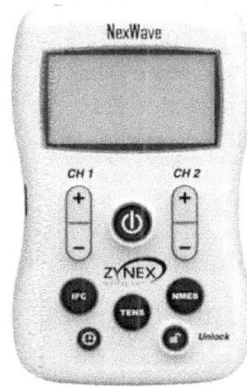

Electrical Muscle Stimulator (EMS)

the NexWave, but similar products by different names are available and basically the same.

Physical Therapy (PT)

Physical therapy after a stroke is designed to help survivors recover as much physical function as possible. Strokes can cause weakness or paralysis, typically on one side of the body, as well as balance, coordination, and movement challenges. The primary goal of physical therapy is to help restore movement and functional abilities in everyday activities such as walking, sitting, standing, and even grasping objects. While the extent of recovery varies depending on the severity of the stroke and how quickly rehabilitation begins, physical therapy often plays a crucial role in regaining lost function. For many stroke survivors, therapy is not only about restoring lost physical abilities but also about rebuilding confidence in their body's capacity to move again (The Stroke Foundation).

One of the main purposes of physical therapists is to assist patients to regain movement, balance, and coordination. Like occupational therapy, assessment testing is administered to evaluate and gauge progress and determine the next steps for continued therapy. Patients are evaluated to determine their abilities and limitations related to efficiently and safely getting in and out of bed, sitting, standing, walking, balance, and a variety of other activities involved with physical movement.

After you've been evaluated, you'll be introduced to a variety of exercises and activities. Let's assume you are wheelchair bound. One of the first things to review is getting to and from the rehab location. I mentioned earlier about taking a bus to rehab, and if you take the bus, the driver will get you situated on the bus. If you do not take the bus and someone is driving you, there's the task of getting in and out of the car. This is one of the first things they will work with you on, although it would have also been reviewed at the rehab hospital. This is one area where the slide board is still used, and you are wearing the gait belt. Yes, you are wearing that gait belt all the time, even at home.

I'm not going to review everything in physical therapy at outpatient therapy because there is a lot. PT sessions move fast, and the therapist had me on my feet and working on taking steps on the first day. I started with using a wide-base cane, then we tried a Hemi walker, which was good, but we did only one day with it and stayed with the cane.

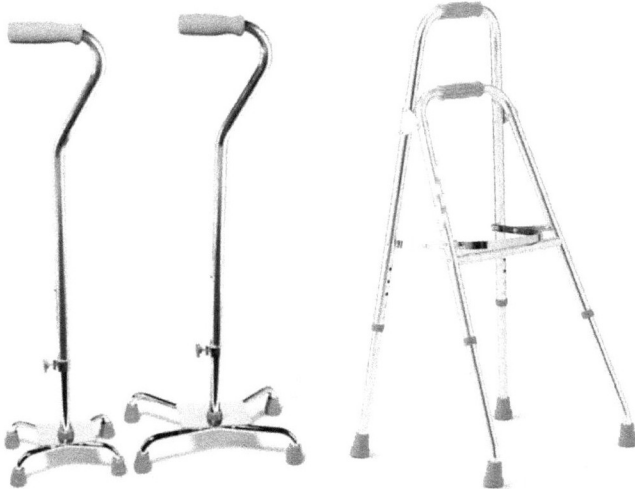

Quad Small & Large Base Cane   Hemi Walker

Using the cane versus the Hemi depends on the patient. The cane will transition to a small base. Due to my progress at the rehab hospital, I was already able to stand briefly and take a few steps with the help of someone holding onto me. You will discover that when learning to walk, every step is difficult. You're fighting with lack of sensation, your knee might buckle, you might not trust your balance, and you might not know where your leg is at, which adds to developing a very bad habit of looking down to watch your foot. You've always got that gait belt on and someone holding onto you with the gait belt. There will come a time when they will not hold onto you—another little thing that feels like a big thing—and a time when you'll be walking for periods of five minutes building up to 15 minutes.

Don't let the size of the therapist fool you. If they happen to have a small build, they are still strong and will not let you fall. Although knowing the therapist will not let you fall does not change the sensation like you're going to fall when you're feeling unstable. Remember, you are retraining your brain as you retrain your muscles and limbs.

On the third day of PT, I had a sudden discomfort, or maybe we can say dislike, for my therapist, Kelsie W. It's difficult to recall the exact emotions. Was I overacting, was I being unreasonable, or was it something else? Whatever it was, I didn't like it. As Kelsie was holding onto me, it felt like with every step, she was tugging, guiding, or nudging me. The next day when she did it again, I smiled and said, "It feels like you're pulling me." She smiled with a little laugh and replied, "That's because I am." Astonished, dismayed, and with I what imagined was a perplexed expression on my face, I looked at her. Kelsie explained the reason for the pulling was because of how patients favor their strong leg, and the tugs are to guide you to put more weight on the weak leg, encouraging a natural step and stride movement. Each tug while you step is training you to trust your weaker leg and build it up.

The explanation combined with additional information made sense. This simple act of a tug or nudge may sound like not a big deal, but that initial experience and emotion can be disruptive and nerve-racking. I would share this story with new patients who I saw having difficulties with their therapists and encourage them to ask their therapist questions instead of feeling frustrated. From that day forward, I loved Kelsie W. and had great respect for her. She also started to incorporate me, or my story, when working with new patients to encourage them to ask questions instead of being frustrated. Why do I call her Kelsie W.? Because there were three therapists named Kelsie—different spellings, but yeah, three of them.

Moving forward, you will work on taking steps and from steps to walking a few feet, which is also where they will have someone following with your wheelchair (aptly named a "wheelchair follow"). As time progresses, you will be given exercises on parallel bars where you practice taking steps and stepping over obstacles. You'll also stand in front of a mirror with a gymnastics bar attached and watch yourself going through various exercises.

As you progress, they will transition you to walking up a step, then multiple steps, and then down steps, which is a significant achievement and brings me to a story I will share with you about one of the patients who, upon being able to walk up the set of stairs and back down, broke down and cried.

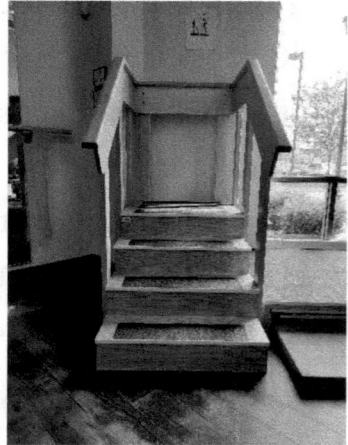

The emotions arrived that day as the patient cried, and you'll see a lot of that as time passes. Do you remember what I said about little things? In physical therapy, a little thing is being able to take one or two steps forward and progress to taking 10 steps, 15 steps, and be able to remain standing for one minute. These are all **little things** but huge achievements.

Most physical therapy facilities are set up to have an area for walking laps. Eventually, you'll be taken on laps. On your first try, you may just take a few steps that will take you a minute or two, and from there, you'll increase the time until you're walking for several minutes, working your way up to five, 10, and 15 minutes. One of the evaluations that are given as you progress is a 15-minute walk to see how far you walk during those 15 minutes, measured in feet.

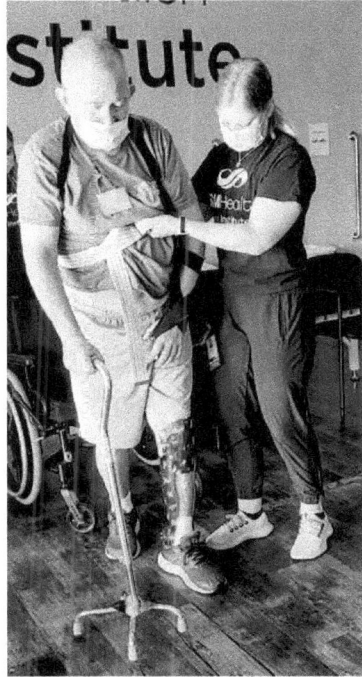

A little thing for me was doing a leg stretch while sitting in the wheelchair. I straightened my leg out on a stool or box, stretched, then repeated the exercise. I had started doing this stretching regularly, and one day the therapist caught me stretching too long and instructed me to stop. I was a little excited and told her I had kept going because I was feeling the pain in the back of my knee and hamstring, and it was not nerve pain, it was the regular type of pain you experience from stretching. This was the first real sensation I had experienced in my left leg, and it was another little thing—real pain, not nerve pain.

Driving and parking a car is something we usually do out of habit, and it's the same with walking—we normally do it without thinking about it. When you're trying to learn how to walk all over again, muscles don't cooperate, and you don't know where your leg or foot is without looking at it. This is something you have to start thinking about, especially when you have a leg that feels like it weighs 100 pounds (remember that heavy leg syndrome mentioned earlier?) and when you try to lift it up, it doesn't go. Instead, you end up flinging it all over the place. I have video evidence of me having that experience. These are more little things that you have to overcome. Another one is figuring out where to plant your foot while you're walking. Planting your foot where you want it to go when you first start taking steps does not work very well. It's not going to go where you want it to go, but in time, you'll be able to move heal to toe like normal.

Leg Brace

You may be prescribed a brace for your leg. If you need a brace, the physical therapist will schedule a fitting. The technical name for the brace is an **AFO**, which stands for **Ankle Foot Orthosis**. A tech will come to the facility, watch and evaluate your walking, and make a cast of your foot and leg. It takes a week or two to receive the brace. The brace makes a significant difference in your ability to stand and walk, and you will notice it right away. Well, maybe not right away, but you will. Like Keanu Reeves said in that *Day the Earth Stood Still* movie: "This body will take some getting used to."

When I was fitted for a brace, there was an option for a design on the brace. I jokingly asked the tech if they did dinosaurs, and he surprised me by answering yes. I got the dinosaurs because the Grandmen were obsessed with dinosaurs.

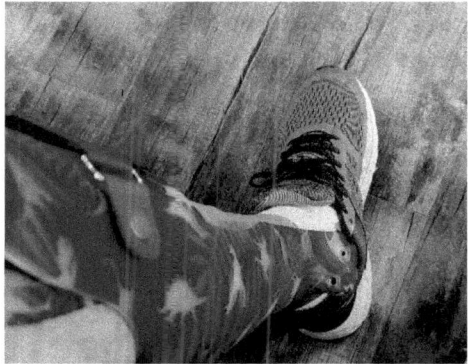

Progression Measured by Little Things

Progress of stroke recovery is measured in inches or feet, not meters or miles. It may be a few weeks or a few months, you'll be sitting there one day with one of the therapists and suddenly you're able to move your pinkie finger, or you're able to touch your pinkie finger with your thumb. Regardless of how long it takes, these are things you couldn't do before. You'll shrug your shoulder, squeeze your shoulder blades, lift your arm out to the side then out front, grasp a ball, raise your knee, stand on one leg. Instead of walking 10 or 15 feet like when you were starting, you're able to walk 150 feet in 15 minutes, and they might even give you a certificate. Several months later, you've progressed to being able to walk 450 feet in 15 minutes. These things are just a few of the accomplishments, the **little things** that add up to **big things**.

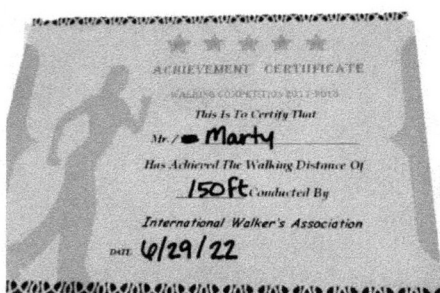

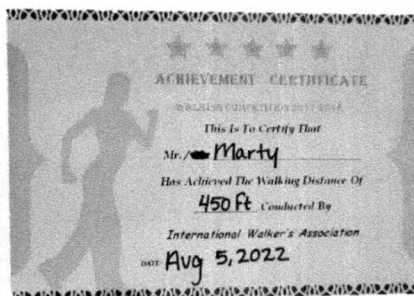

Before I went to outpatient therapy, I discovered little things happening at the rehab hospital. Most significant was the night I was able to move my left foot, or at least, it felt like I was moving it. I felt like I was wiggling my toes, but when I looked, no wiggling was happening, but my mind was preparing for the wiggling. Within a few nights, I was able to slightly move my foot, which was one of my first little things, and it was accompanied by nerve pain. The nerve pain can be slight but could be severe.

Walking, Talking, and Chewing Gum

I use this analogy to illustrate the task of having to do more than one thing at a time when learning how to walk again. As I progressed from one minute to five minutes to 10 minutes and so on, the one thing I had to focus on was one step at a time. I would not have been able to talk and chew gum, but as I progressed, I was able to talk as I walked while simultaneously focusing on the step, heel to toe, combined with the cane placement. A lot of little actions are involved with just taking a step, which will become evident as you progress.

Smiles and Chuckles

One thing I can positively state is I have maintained a positive attitude...well, most of the time. I tried to always smile even when there were aches, pain, discomfort, or nerve pain. You'll become aware that we all grimace. I would grimace with a smile, and I would chuckle when it hurt. In outpatient therapy when I saw other patients grimacing, I would smile and tell them to smile and chuckle too. As the months passed, I was often told that my positivity inspired others.

Grimace with a smile and chuckle when it hurts.

I developed a habit of telling patients how good they were doing or looking. I did so with enthusiasm and an assortment of words and made-up words:

- Fantabulous
- Fantabalistic
- Phenomenal
- Phenomenos
- Supercalifragilistic
- Fragilistic
- Unbelievable
- Unbelievably awesome
- Absolutely astonishing
- Astonishingly impressive
- Remarkably inspiring
- Wonderful
- Tremendous
- Magnificent
- Extraordinary
- Beautifully Splendid
- And many many more

I know I've said it over and over about having a positive attitude. Attitudes are contagious, and my so-called words of wisdom to you are to maintain positivity, smile, and chuckle. Maintain a positive focus and perspective, be resilient, and inspire others with your courage and never-give-up attitude.

Why Does It Hurt So Much? Too Many Prayers

When other patients would ask, "Why does it hurt so much?" I would joke, "Too many prayers!" I would explain that all the prayers were working because if we're feeling things, feeling pain and nerve pain, that means our body is doing its repair work—and repair work is good. I equated our recovery to computer hardware and software updates, and on my website, I sell T-shirts with the phrase "Software Update in Progress."

Observing Success

During your time at outpatient therapy, you will notice other patients' improvements and the emotional excitement experienced over little things like being able to move a finger or stand up at a table.

I'm getting off track here to share one such observation. There was an 18-year-old girl I will call Elle, who was a patient. She had symptoms similar to a stroke with arm and leg paralysis, but her condition was not caused by a stroke. During a session, Elle was given the task of attempting to stand up independently out of her wheelchair at a table. After some grimaces, smiles, and chuckles, she did it. She placed her hands on the table and stood up. Her face expressed the difficulty in making that stand, but also projected a sense of accomplishment. The therapist, another therapist nearby, and I were a little overwhelmed with pride for her completing that task. It can be very emotional to witness someone else's achievements and, again, one of those little things. Even now as I write this about Elle, the memory makes me emotional.

Resistance to Change

We may all be set in our ways, especially us older individuals, but the time has come for us to not resist change. I mention this because as the months go by, we train ourselves to do things differently, and then one day, a therapist will start moving us in another direction, such as getting kicked out of your wheelchair. Every day you have rolled in and rolled out of the outpatient therapy facility, and suddenly one day, they say, "Start walking in, no more wheelchair." The daily routine of rolling from one session to another, one place to another, including the restroom, all of a sudden stops. Now you walk to all those places. Someone will walk with you, and you walk slowly and carefully, but you will be walking.

That wheelchair may have become a crutch that you are resistant to give up, and if I'm being honest, that's how I felt. I joked about feeling I was being punished and not being allowed to roll all over the place like a toddler crawling around. I got over it, and the new instruction pushed me to do more. Each change forces you to become more self-dependent. You may still need to use the wheelchair but not all the time. I've often mentioned that your situation may be different, and you may end up walking in a shorter period of time or a longer period of time. I have seen several patients who were in wheelchairs when they started outpatient therapy and walked out in a full stride on their graduation day.

Don't resist change.
It's not just recovery and
rehabilitation, it's the rest of your life.

OUTPATIENT THERAPY NEARING ITS END

Discharge or an end to outpatient therapy generally ends in one of three ways. One is when outpatient therapy is no longer helping you progress. The other transition from physical therapy is graduation, where they've done everything they could for you, you've made significant progress, and you walk out with congratulations on your recovery. The unfortunate third reason, at least in the United States, is insurance, and I bring this up primarily for those who have Medicare Advantage Plans.

If you have **Medicare Advantage Plans**, you may want to read this next section, but if you carry different insurance, you may jump ahead to the next section.

Insurance

DISCLAIMER: I am not an insurance expert, and the views I mention on Medicare Advantage Plans are my opinion based on personal experience and discussions with other patients.

The unfortunate third reason for discharge from outpatient therapy is insurance. This became a frustration of mine as I witnessed patients who were making progress but were kicked out of therapy by their insurance. "Kicked Out" is a harsh term that is not liked or used by therapists and administrators. It is emotional for them when they are notified that one of their patients is being discharged. However, "kicked out" was the preferred phrase used by patients themselves who were discharged because their Medicare Advantage Plan did not approve continued outpatient therapy.

Right now, some of you might be thinking about all the negative things you've heard about Medicare and how bad Medicare is. Well, surprise, it's NOT Medicare with the bad rep but the insurance companies that offer the Medicare Advantage Plans. Yes, those pesky Advantage Plans that scam, con, and prey on seniors (in my opinion) with too-good-to-be-true benefits. Yes, they will give you a free gym membership, but what if you get hurt at the gym and you need physical therapy, will they cover it and for how long?

During my time in outpatient therapy, I had conversations with about half a dozen patients who were discharged because of their Advantage Plans. These patients were progressing exceptionally well, and it seemed they were only in outpatient therapy for a few months. On one occasion, we saw two therapists in a corner with a patient consoling her as she was crying her eyes out because she was notified it was her last day due to her Advantage Plan would not cover her continued therapy.

My wife and I learned a lesson about Advantage Plans a few years earlier when our mom, who was in an assisted living facility, was taken to the hospital. The doctor prescribed physical therapy, and it was denied by the Advantage Plan she had. I inquired as to why, and the administrator of the hospital and similarly the administrator of the assisted living facility both explained that if she had not been on an Advantage Plan, then her Medicare and Medicaid would have covered it. They both said this was a regular occurrence and saw it all the time. They suggested we cancel the Advantage Plan immediately to avoid future care denials. We canceled it, and a few months later during another hospital stay for our mom, physical therapy was prescribed and was approved by Medicare.

As I finish my rant about insurance, it is important to point out that there is a difference between an Advantage Plan and a supplement plan, and my suggestion is to do your research, ask the what-if questions, and not necessarily listen to friends suggesting Advantage Plans, which is how our mom arrived at getting an Advantage Plan.

I apologize for this digression about insurance, but the purpose of this book is to pass on information I've learned through my experience and those I've been in rehab with so you can be better prepared. This, unfortunately, was too common of an occurrence for me not to mention it.

TRANSITION FROM OUTPATIENT THERAPY

After ten months of five days a week in outpatient therapy, the day arrived for my official discharge, otherwise known as graduation. The staff makes a big deal out of graduation for patients. Many of the staff and therapists get attached to the patients, and a few tears may be shed on the way out the door.

Life is about to change again, just like the day when it all started. The end of the routine of going to outpatient therapy every day—whether it had been a few months, six months, or ten months—is another transition you have to face. It is important to maintain the same activity and exercise level, or even to increase it.

Don't make the mistake of slowing down!

Adjustments

It's okay to take a break, but there may be a temptation to slow down permanently and not do as much walking and exercises. Adjusting to a new daily routine may unintentionally result in less activity, even though it's just as needed as when you were in outpatient therapy. It's important to be mindful of how much you're doing or not doing.

I'll admit and say that it is easy to fall into new routines that interfere with what should be the priority of walking and doing exercises. As a few months passed after graduation from outpatient therapy, I noticed a decrease in my walking endurance, coupled with upper body spasticity that slowed me down. In hindsight, I realize that if I had kept up my activity level, I may not have experienced those regressions.

Squirrels in Our Heads

When I see someone having a bad day, in a bad mood, or depressed, I will sometimes joke with them about squirrels running around in their head. We all have squirrels that run around in our heads, and sometimes it's not like regular squirrels, but big rabid squirrels that create distractions, interfering with what we would normally be doing or thinking. You have to get rid of those rabid squirrels and maintain your positive attitude. Don't give depression the opportunity to nest in your head. When a squirrel starts running around in your head, try thinking about Doug the dog in the animated movie *Up* (see, another movie reference), and hopefully the image of Doug being distracted by a squirrel will make you smile, then you'll be in the right frame of mind to get back on track.

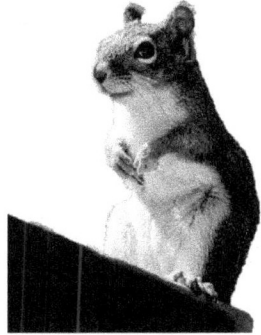

Train for Life

I mentioned earlier that life as you knew it has changed, and as the months passed, I became aware of this again and again. I developed a philosophy of sorts that the change would introduce me to new outlooks, and one of those outlooks was the concept of "train for life." This new challenge we have been given is not temporary; it is permanent for most of us, and our approach needs to be a "train for life" approach, a complete change from how we used to do things. Similar to how runners, swimmers, and many other athletes train every day, not just during the sport's season but throughout the year. Regardless of if you were in poor health or good health before the stroke, you're still faced with moving forward, and I encourage you to adopt a train-for-life approach.

TRAIN FOR LIFE

NAVIGATE THE OBSTACLES THAT
LIFE CHALLENGES YOU WITH

OVERCOME THOSE OBSTACLES

BE A FIGHTER

BE AN INSPIRATION FOR OTHERS

ALWAYS MAINTAIN A POSITIVE AND
OPTIMISTIC ATTITUDE

STAY STRONG

EMBRACE LIFE

MORE OTHER THINGS

I mentioned earlier "A Few Other Things": the Fatigue Factor, Nerve Pain, Spasms, and Spasticity. Here I present *more* "Other Things" you might want to keep in mind.

Weird Feelings

Muscle stretch versus nerve pain: As time passes, you may notice nerve pain subsiding when exercising or walking. Tapping, lifting, holding, or other movement of the paralyzed arm and leg will cause nerve pain, and while it may be difficult to fully explain, there is a difference between muscle pain and nerve pain, and you'll need to distinguish the difference. If I'm being honest, you'll experience a lot of weird feelings, and the best way of explaining it is simply saying it's *weird*.

The Sensations—It's Not a Music Group

In the days and weeks after the stroke, you will experience a variety of sensations, some of which cannot really be explained. The most common is a lack of touch sensation even while there is what the doctors would call pressure sensation. For example, if I am grasping something, I know I am holding it, like holding on to a grab bar or a bottle. I know I'm holding on to an object without the benefit of touch—the touch sensation is nonexistent—but I do experience a pressure sensation. However, you have to pay attention when holding something because if you forget for a second, then you may drop the object or lose your grip.

One of the things that therapists will do is tap you on the back of the knee or other parts of your body to signal to your brain to react and move. Therefore, you can feel a tap and know somebody's tapping you. I would advise you to pay attention when you're washing your hands or in a shower because while you may not have touch sensation, you do have sensitivity to hot and cold, and the first time you notice it, you may experience an owie reaction. The therapist may also have you work on grasping marbles, balls, and an assortment of small objects to work on dexterity as well as this touch sensation. I often did a zombie voice of "brains, braines" when the therapist brought the bucket of blue brains to me to work on.

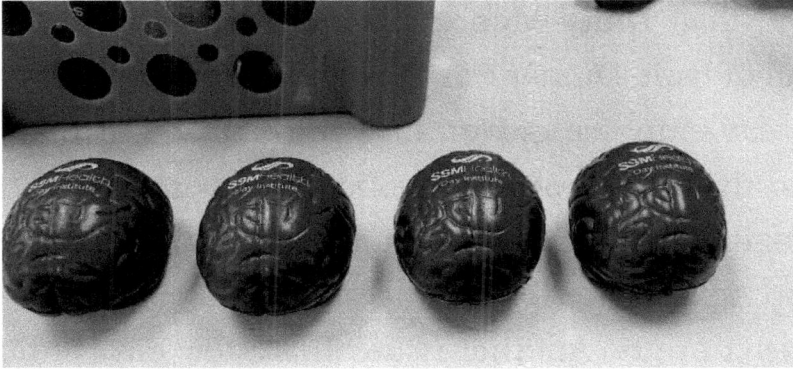

Medications

There is an array of medications the doctors may have you on, especially if you are diabetic. My first bad reaction to a medication was after going home from the hospital. The diabetic medication metformin turned out to be a problem for me. In the hospital, they had me on a sliding scale of insulin and changed that to metformin when I left. I mentioned earlier having the car sickness on the way to outpatient therapy my first day. Within days of going home from the hospital, I experienced a problem eating—or rather, not eating.

At the rehabilitation hospital, I was on a good diet and eating well; however, within a day of going home, something was happening. I'd have about half a protein shake or piece of bread or biscuit for breakfast, and for lunch, I'd eat peanut butter snack crackers or the small Dinty Moore chicken dumplings cup or a cup of fruit. Dinner was the bigger problem. I was able to eat soup, ice cream, or a milkshake, but that was mostly it. Attempts to eat solid foods were futile. I tried grazing with little success and had to have a red Solo cup next to me for an uncontrollable gag reflex that wasn't pretty. Another issue after a few days at home was no bowel movements.

A few weeks later, I saw my primary care doctor. We discussed what was going on, and he proceeded to tell me that it made sense because in addition to diabetes, metformin was used as a weight loss medication. Turned out, my A1C and blood sugar levels had lowered, and the metformin was doing its weight loss job. The doctor took me off the metformin and did not replace it because I was now considered prediabetic status. As for the bowel movements, which I hadn't had for 14 days, the doctor said given my liquid diet, it was not surprising. Still, he sent me to get an ultrasound just to be sure.

The ultrasound revealed no problems. After stopping the metformin, it took a couple days for my appetite and everything to return. I was able to start eating a small breakfast; usually in the car on the way to rehab, we'd drive through Chick-fil-A and get nuggets. On school days, it was routine for the Grandmen to drive to rehab with us to drop me off and then they'd go to school. Sometimes they'd walk me in.

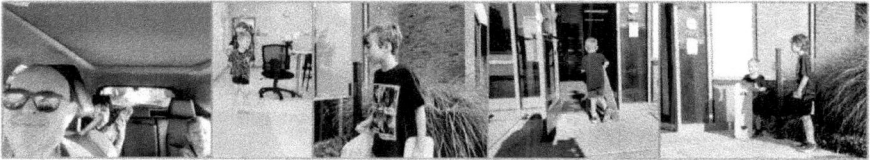

As for other medications, your doctor may have you on others for other health-related reasons. Experiencing spasms, especially at night, is common, and there are two commonly prescribed medications for stroke patients for spasticity. The first one I was on was gabapentin, which is used to help control spasms or partial seizures. Discussions at rehab among patients offered mixed opinions about gabapentin, with some saying it worked while for some of us it did not work. My neurologist changed the gabapentin to baclofen, a medication used to treat muscle spasticity. The baclofen was taken three times daily and seemed to work for me, although I still experienced nighttime spasms, just not as severe. A side effect of baclofen was lightheadedness and one of those weird feelings I've mentioned. I had to cut back and eventually stopped taking it (with doctor approval).

Botox

Botox is not for everyone. Eight months after the stroke and several months of outpatient therapy, I was making continual progress and improvement in walking with the cane; movement of my hand, wrist, elbow, and shoulder; dexterity and so on. However, I was still experiencing spasticity that caused tightness of the muscles, ligaments, and joints. The ability to extend the elbow completely was nonexistent, and for the most part, the elbow remained at a 90-degree angle. After a stroke, you will likely spend a lot of time doing your own research to find things that may help you. One of the topics I found was Botox. A few patients I knew who received Botox found it helpful, while others did not.

I discussed Botox with the occupational therapist, and she felt that it might be time to talk with my neurologist. I made an appointment, and the therapist accompanied me to the appointment. She and the doctor talked using all the medical terminology, which sounded a lot like a foreign language, or Klingon to me, but it was educational. We decided to do the Botox.

On your visit to the neurologist, I would suggest wearing shorts and a T-shirt to allow easy access to the injection areas. The doctor discussed the affected areas with the spasticity. It was interesting and encouraging as I told him what I was experiencing and he knew exactly what I was referring to, and it seemed like he was reading my mind as he politely finished some of my sentences as I described my experiences.

The Botox procedure was not complicated. I remained in the wheelchair, and the doctor applied a dab of gel and electrodes to a few spots on my leg, thigh, and arm. The electrode connected to a machine that had a monitor. Next, he prepared the syringe. He placed a thin cover over the needle that had a wire connection to the machine. As he started to make the first injection, the monitor lit up with a bunch of squiggly lines going up and down. The injection is not like a regular shot because the doctor watches

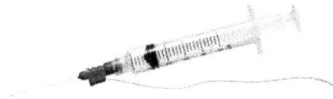

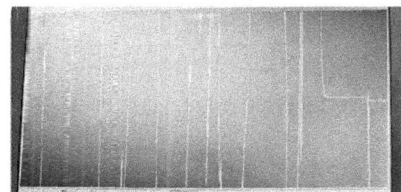

EMG (electromyography) Monitor

the monitor as he guides the needle to the right spot, so this takes about thirty seconds, give or take. The injection is repeated for each area, so for me, it was four to six places. Since the area being injected was in the bad arm and leg, I didn't feel the stick of the needle, although during later visits, I occasionally felt a slight stick, but nothing dramatic.

There are several types of machines or methods neurologists use to guide the injections. Sonagram is one and my neurologist utilized EMG (electromyography). EMG is used in Botox injections to precisely locate the target muscle by monitoring its electrical activity, allowing for a more accurate placement of the needle and ensuring the Botox is injected directly into the desired muscle, particularly important for treating conditions like muscle spasms or dystonia where precise muscle targeting is crucial; essentially, EMG acts as a guide to ensure the injection is delivered in the most effective location (Klein, 1998).

It is amazing to watch the procedure on the monitor. It reminded me of the *Matrix* movie scenes with all the numbers flowing across the screen. You may have noticed by now that I make a lot of references to movies—a favorite pastime of mine.

Within a week, I had less pain in my hip flexor, and I experienced significant improvement in the range of motion of my arm and hip. I have continued to get

Botox every 90 days, and it has significantly helped improve my range of motion, and I've also noticed reduced nerve pain associated with stretching. Just keep in mind that even though Botox worked for me, it may not for you.

Posture Problem

The tendency to lean forward and look at the ground when walking may not be noticeable at first but over time can develop into a bad habit. A year later when you are out somewhere, you may see your reflection in a store window and be surprised to see yourself leaning forward—and not just leaning forward but exaggeratedly way forward. One of the medical terms for this is known as forward head posture (FHP). This is something that can be corrected with strengthening and stretching exercises, chiropractic care, physical therapy, and posture training. Something else I noticed was when I attempted to stand straight, I felt as if I might fall backward. I attribute this to occasional balance issues and the body being accustomed to leaning forward. I will discuss the benefits of having a trainer in a later section, and this is another area a trainer can provide help with.

Walkers, Canes, and Buggies, Oh My!

Hemi Walker and Cane

During your time at therapy, you're likely to have been introduced to a Hemi walker and a variety of canes, including one with a quad wide base and one with a small base. At first I tried a Hemi one-arm walker that worked well; however, I transitioned to a quad cane, which has a four-point base, after a few days. I've been using the quad small base, which has worked well for me.

After I was out of therapy and as time passed, I experimented with some equipment to help me improve my walking. When the spasticity had slowed me down so much, there came a point when I wanted to experiment with anything that might help.

Upright Rollator Walker

One experiment was an upright rollator walker, which at the time, I felt made sense. I think an upright walker can be beneficial; however, my results are not typical. Initially, the upright walker worked great, and even the trainer thought it

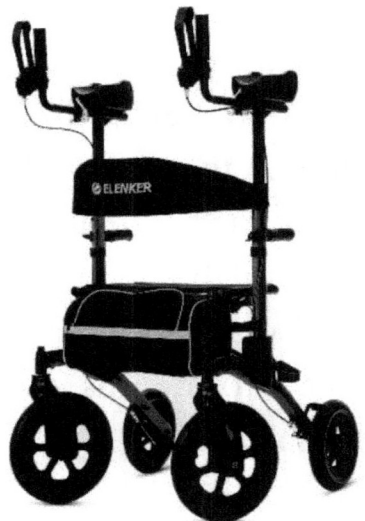

was working with no negative effects. The first few days using the walker seemed good, with only one issue in my left upper body. An initial arm stiffness made it a bit difficult, but I was persistent and made it work. I was doing 10- to 15-minute walks the first few days and only experienced some upper body tightness. I noticed that after I was off the walker, the upper body spasticity intensified and extended to the leg. This occurred for the first week, and at the time, it made sense that this new or different exercise would cause this.

I continued to use the walker for about another six weeks or so, including with the trainer, but unfortunately, the issue continued. While initially my use of the walker was good, as the weeks passed, my pace was decreasing. During sessions with the trainer, we noticed that the slow pace I was walking at with a cane prior to using the walker was diminishing further, and the upper body spasticity was worsening. The heaviness of the arm and leg I was experiencing was also feeling heavier.

The trainer noted that I was visibly behind where I was prior to starting the walker, and the increased tightness of the upper body was interfering with my progress in the therapy and exercises for the upper body. We decided to alter the experiment and not use the walker for a week and then a second week.

The results were perplexing, to say the least, and my initial reaction was that I had wasted two months experimenting, setting me back months in my progress. However, after switching back to the cane, the spasticity had reduced, and I was able to walk much better with the cane at an improved pace. The overall tightness and heaviness were reduced. We concluded I was an anomaly of sorts, although spasticity was the culprit and not the upright walker. I think each of us is different, and the upright walker could be a great tool to help with walking depending on your individual situation.

Rollator Walker

I tried a rollator walker, otherwise known as a buggy. Keep in mind that the therapist will not recommend or allow you to use one because of safety and other concerns. The first time I tried one, it did not work so well because I could not get a grip of the handle with my left hand. The flexion of my arm and

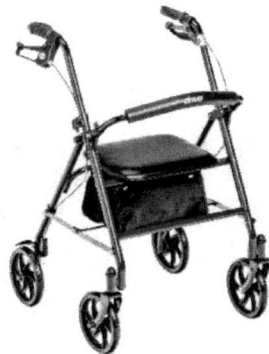

hand did not cooperate; however, a year later, after a lot of improvement with arm spasticity, I tried it again with success, but I got rid of it and kept with cane.

The ultimate goal would be to not have to use any canes or walkers, or even a wheelchair, but our reality is that we may have to continue to use something. Again, this all depends on our individual circumstances.

Elliptical Recumbent Bike

When I had breaks at outpatient therapy, I used what they called the "stepper." The official name is a recumbent cross trainer, which I liked using, and I would do 10 to 20 minutes of peddling on it. My left

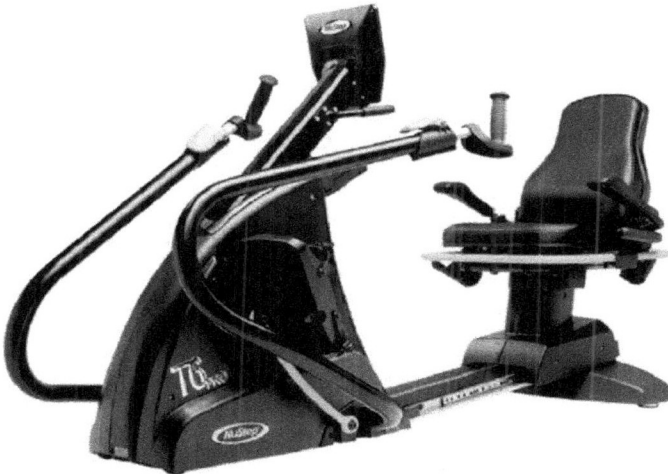

Recumbent Cross Trainer used at Outpatient Therapy

arm was still very tight, and I had difficulty with grip and angle, which prevented me from holding on to the handle, so I just peddled.

After I had been home about six months, I ordered an elliptical recumbent bike, which would be a similar

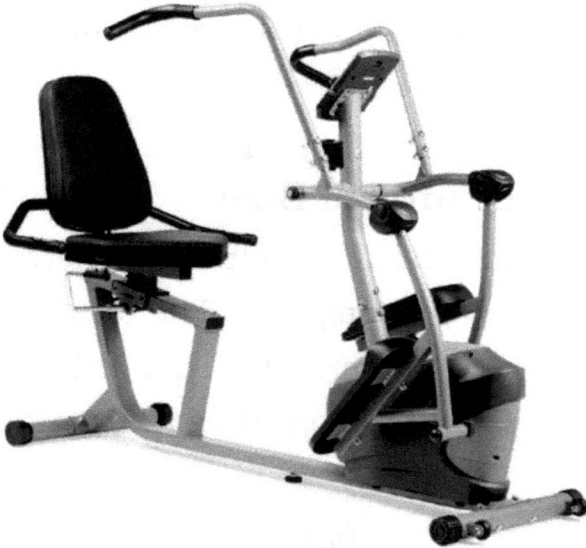

Sunny Health & Fitness Compact Performance Recumbent Bike

machine. These machines go by many names and varying prices. I looked for something that would work the arms and legs, and something that would fit in our apartment. The first one I ordered I had to return because it was too big.

There are standard stationary bicycle-type machines, but the benefit of the elliptical types is they provide added motion versus just peddling. The handles on this type of machine allowed me to work on grip while having full motion, back and forth, for the arms, which helped significantly with stretching all the upper body muscles while also using a slight wrist movement. The first week I experienced nerve and stretch pain in the upper body, but after a week, it was gone. Pay attention to the weak leg as that knee tends to fall out to the side, but this just takes awareness and making the necessary adjustment.

Ideal Stretch Hamstring & Calf Stretcher

As far as more other things go, this is one my trainer introduced me to. The trainer was planning on retiring, and she suggested the Ideal Stretch Original. This was a device I could use by myself to stretch the calves and hamstrings, and it works.

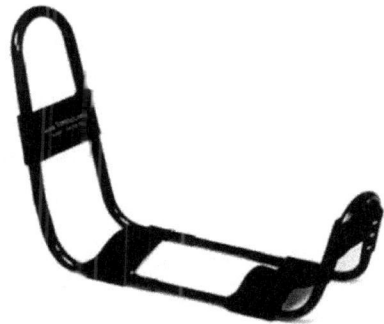

Hamstring & Calf Stretcher

Hand Spasticity

Hand spasticity is probably something that you'll experience. This is a common condition that can occur after a stroke, affecting around one in four stroke survivors. It's caused by disrupted connections between the brain and the hand muscles, which can lead to increased muscle tone and stiffness. This can make it difficult to move the hands or fingers or grasp objects (Lee 2021, How to Manage Hand Spasticity).

I had hand spasticity, and working the hand was a continuous necessity to prevent the condition from getting worse. Since the hand is connected to the arm and all the ligaments and muscles are connected, the hand spasticity contributed to that upper body spasticity problem.

My hand and fingers curled inward; some days it would be worse than others. A conversation with the trainer relating to remedies for the hand spasticity would turn out to be one of those "Duh" moments. During the conversation, which took place almost two years after the stroke, the trainer mentioned, "What about a hand brace?" This was one of the many things, in hindsight, I wished I'd known or realized sooner.

I did some research and ordered a hand brace. I started with a "carpal tunnel wrist brace." This one had metal rods in it that helped keep the wrist straight, and it worked fine for a while; however, I noticed the fingers would still curl inward and, except for the wrist, I was still

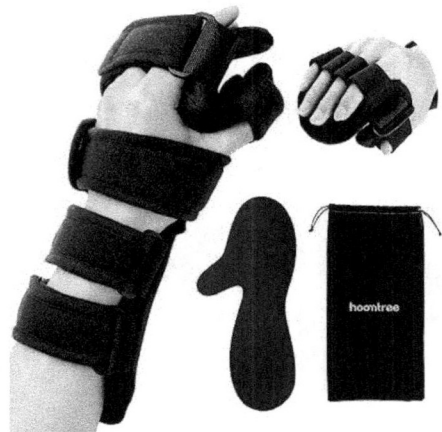

having the spasticity problems. The next one I ordered, and still use, was a "stroke resting hand splint." This one worked great and is designed to keep the hand at its natural position. At first it felt weird, but after a few minutes, things calmed down. I found that wearing this a few hours or longer a day seemed to stop progression of the hand spasticity while reducing or helping the upper body spasticity. How did it help? Everything is connected, and a lot less of those ligaments and muscles were tightening. This happened gradually over time, but the splint definitely helped, and as for hindsight, I would have gotten the splint much sooner than later.

Prior to getting the hand splint, I did try one of those robotic hand gloves, and while the advertisements looked good and I'm sure it works for some people, it did not for me. I'll admit, I may have been short on patience trying to use it. Putting it on was burdensome, and once turned on, it was distracting if I tried to do anything, and I got tired of it quickly.

The Value of a Trainer

A year or so before my stroke, a friend of mine, David, a writer and karate instructor, broke his ankle.

He had surgery and went through recovery and physical therapy, but his doctor told him he would probably never be able to do the karate-type activities like he used to. That conversation got him thinking, and so he found a trainer. A year later, he posted on Facebook that he was 100% recovered, thanks to his trainer. He was able to perform and teach karate at the same level he had previously been able to do before he broke his ankle.

A few weeks prior to my discharge from outpatient therapy, I recalled David's experience and decided to research trainers. Aside from being reputable and experienced, the main criteria I had was finding a trainer who had familiarity with stroke victims. Familiarity is important because, frankly, a lot happens within the body after a stroke, and one wrong stretch, bend, or turn could be painful and damaging. I cannot emphasize enough how important it is that a trainer understands the physiology involved with things like spasticity.

I contacted the company that David had used, a franchise of GYMGUYZ, and I'd recommend them. They set me up with an experienced trainer named Barb, who had previous qualifications as a physical therapist and extensive experience with stroke victims and people with various physical disabilities. Barb was the right choice for me. Within the first two sessions,

Barb surprised me as I noticed her using terminology I'd heard in outpatient therapy, plus it was apparent she understood what I was experiencing and how to approach it.

Why a Trainer

There are many reasons to hire a trainer to help. Combating spasticity is a big one, plus assisting with maintaining forward progress with strength building, range of motion, and the other accomplishments made during outpatient therapy. The major issue with spasticity is the tightening of ligaments and joints, and while Botox injections might help relieve some of the spasticity and associated pain, it does not eliminate it. Someone who knows what they're doing can help with working on the areas experiencing spasticity.

Two years after the stroke, I still worked with the trainer, and every session I still experienced a little nerve pain from different stretches and manipulation of joints and ligaments, but as time has passed, I have less and less or no nerve pain at all, and the range of motion has improved tremendously. Still, that Saber tooth tiger of a hip flexor muscle needs stretching, along with other areas. This is important because the affected side of the body's arm and leg need attention; otherwise, the tightness and constricting of ligaments and joints could intensify, causing more severe spasticity.

I am not suggesting that you must get a trainer—it's not a necessity—but there is a positive benefit. Barb provided a wealth of educational information, not to mention introducing a variety of exercises and different approaches to dealing with setbacks and spasticity.

A big plus to a trainer is the feedback and encouragement they supply. Spasticity has been a constant battle for me in my arm and upper body, where constricting of muscles happen that talk to my leg, making it difficult to walk sometimes. Encouragement helps. Also, at times, a trainer will notice little things like *posture*, bending a knee, bending a hip, lowering the arm, or dozens of other little things that we're not aware of or pay attention to, but we need to be reminded about what could be corrected. All of this helps you maintain focus that you need to work every day.

Retrain your brain!

Spasticity interferes with our sensory skills. **Sensory integration** was explained by my trainer to help me better understand why attempting a movement may not work or why the arm or leg does something we did not intentionally want it to do, like the foot making a sudden outward jerking motion.

Sensory integration is a term that has been used to describe processes in the brain that allow us to take information we receive from our senses, organize it, and respond appropriately. The process in the brain needs to be retrained to allow us to take the signals from our senses, make sense of those signals, and respond appropriately. An example could be when you are walking, focused on the placement of your foot, and you forget about your arm for a moment; your subconscious thinks that your arm is doing what it naturally would be doing, swinging by your side. The new reality might be that the arm is not swinging and instead tends to kind of drift forward, helped by the heaviness of the arm, and suddenly giving you a sensation of falling forward that you compensate for. You may think your arm is straight by your side, but it's not. The hand and lower arm are out front, and you find you need to place your hand on your lower waist and hold it against you to keep the awareness of where your arm is. When you work with a trainer, they would help with noticing things that you need to retrain and how to improve your overall range of motion and sensory awareness.

If you have the financial resources, I strongly recommend a personal trainer. You can also go to fitness centers or gyms. Just make sure that anyone who helps you is aware of your condition. You can easily hurt yourself without knowing it or feeling it. When you try new exercises or a machine in a gym, the spasticity monster might scream at you—and not necessarily when you are using the machine or doing the exercise, but as soon as you stop or minutes later. Always be careful when trying something new.

HINDSIGHT EPIPHANIES AND GOALS

Set yourself up for success—not failure.

As I draw closer to finishing up, I've found that the more I write, the more I remember. With the benefit of hindsight, there are a lot of lessons learned. You'll probably experience it too, having those "duh" moments you wished you thought of sooner. It might be something like how you get in and out of the shower or how you go to the bathroom, get in and out of bed, put your socks on, or get dressed. With trial and error, you discover different angels, twists, turns, steps, and an assortment of ways that make it easier to accomplish tasks. With each discovery, you tap yourself on the head, shake your head, laugh a bit, and think about how simple it was and wish you had thought of it sooner.

You may experience, as I did, setbacks or slowing down. Spasticity can be the main problem causing a setback. Heaviness in your leg and upper body tends to slow down your ability to walk with a stride and instead take one step at a time. The heaviness causes you to slow down. The bigger issue for me was the heaviness of the upper body, which I equate to a toddler hanging around your neck, therefore causing a balancing issue. You learn to compensate for this, and some days the heaviness is less bothersome.

When you're tired and it hurts, it's easy for someone to tell you to "work through the pain" and "suck it up." You may not like it, but that's what you have to do, you must do.

Energy Suck—that's what I've called it. Sometimes when I take a step, and with every step after it, I get an energy drain. For anyone who's a parent and you've lost your kid for a second, you feel what we call your heart sinking; it hits your stomach, and you feel the energy drain from your core, and that is the best way I can explain the energy drain or suck you feel as a stroke survivor. It's annoying and frustrating, and why it happens, I can't explain, other than it happens.

Goals

We all have different goals depending on our perceived limitations. However, as I've said before, our biggest obstacle, our biggest limitation, is our attitude. With a positive attitude, we can do it, whatever the "it" might be. Walk again, even if limited, doing things with the affected hand, even if not at 100%, we are still able to get the task done. Of course we have physical limits, but with perseverance and a positive attitude, we can complete the task.

Debbie had a bit of inspiration and a vision in a dream. She told me that she saw me rucking and gave me the goal of rucking again. Now, all of you military types know what I'm talking about and might have just let out an enthusiastic "Yeaaaah," or something to that effect.

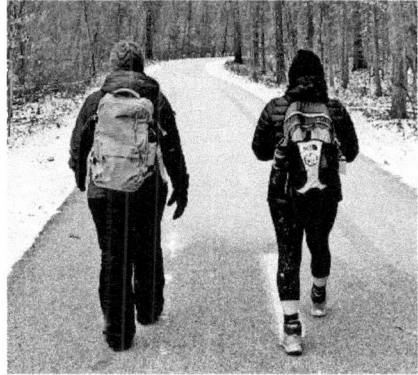

If you do not know, the nonmilitary definition for rucking is walking while carrying a heavy weight in a backpack. The rucksack is a military backpack that we'd carry equipment in, weighing 50-plus pounds. It was a regular routine to go rucking a few times a week for an hour or so.

There it is: A goal to go rucking again.

During the editing process of this book, I mentioned this part to Debbie, and she lightheartedly told me that it wasn't a dream, it was a "premonition." I liked how she put that. It gave me another mental approach to my recovery: Visualize your goals. Visualize yourself doing those goals.

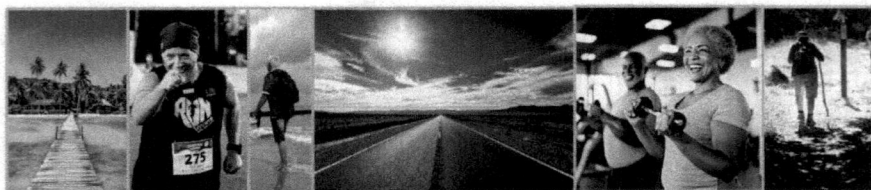

Visualize Your Goals

You may not have a goal to go rucking, but you can have a goal, and "rucking" can be interchangeable with anything you'd want to do. There's no such thing as too many goals; you can never have too many goals, too many dreams, or too many aspirations. You can, however, have too many reasons or excuses to not try, to not care, to quit.

Don't come up with reasons why you can't.
Come up with the reasons why you can.

A Not-So-Happy Ending

I imagine the title of this section got your attention, which was on purpose to make a point that there will be setbacks, and if you do not experience a setback, that's good for you. I've covered a lot, and you will likely learn a lot more as you progress. There will be setbacks, hiccups, and bad days.

Don't let the bad days win!

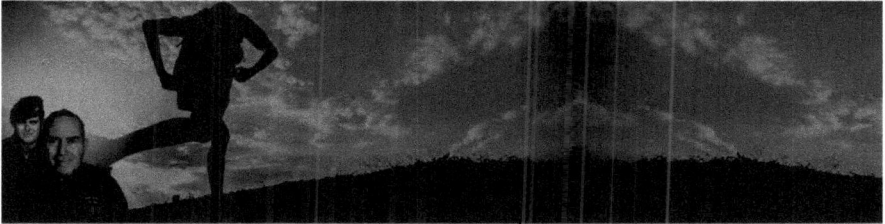

Don't Let The Bad Days Win

I already mentioned that you are a death-dodging stroke survivor, and if your ailment is something different, substitute the word "stroke" with your ailment and be positive, strong, and don't give up. You can learn from others and inspire others with your positivity and success.

Returning to Outpatient Therapy

Setbacks happen, and marathon races happen. The vast majority of marathon participants are not in the race to win. They are in it to be in it, to accomplish a goal, to achieve something, and know that they trained and did their best to participate in their race. As stroke victims, we must participate in our own metaphorical marathon. Regardless of illness, stroke, cancer, or whatever life sends our way, we must be active participants in our marathon and not let setbacks stop us, discourage us, enable us, or make us quit.

Months after I left outpatient therapy, I experienced a gradual decline in my mobility and my ability to walk. Truthfully, I did not notice it right away, and it was more like six months to a year before I was fully aware of it. The reason for the decline was my own fault as I kept myself busy on various projects—remember about keeping your mind busy— and in doing that, I reduced the amount of time I spent walking and doing physical activities. I was still working with the trainer and doing my own exercises, but the reality was, I moved less and I declined.

I was trying to do a variety of physical things in an effort to improve and maintain my mobility, but I felt I was not improving. I discussed this with my neurologist and asked him about returning to physical therapy for an evaluation and tune-up of sorts. My intent for trying physical therapy again was that the therapist could provide a new approach to activities that I would incorporate into my daily routine. I was evaluated and attended physical therapy for a short period and changed my daily routine.

This is where I emphasize, emphasize, and reemphasize the absolute necessity to NOT let yourself slow down. You must "train for life" and do whatever physical activities are recommended and necessary for your situation.

I could joke and tell you that I purposely slowed down so that I could share a lesson with you about slowing down. I did not slow down on purpose, but it happened—don't let it happen to you!

Don't be upset by the results you didn't get
from the work you did not do.

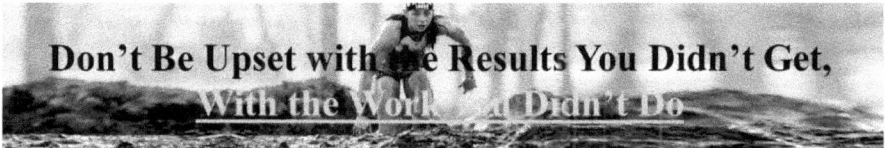

Don't Be Upset with the Results You Didn't Get, With the Work that Didn't Do

Strokes Don't Discriminate

Most people walk around and think, "It won't happen to me," be it a stroke, heart attack, cancer, heart disease, or death. A lot of us walk around and do not take care of the temple of our bodies we've been given. Smokers smoke, drug users use, the overweight stay overweight, the overeaters overeat, and the list can go on relating to some of the preventive things that we *can* do something about. If you don't like what I just said, that's okay, and I'll admit I was one of the "it won't happen to me" people; however, I made a change and you can too...before change is forced on you.

All the bad things that can happen to us don't discriminate. I use celebrities to illustrate my point. A large segment of society has a fascination with celebrities, so much so that fans elevate celebrities to indestructible superhero status, and yet, even celebrities have bad things happen to them, even strokes. Here's a few famous names who have suffered from a stroke:

Hailey Bieber, Emelia Clarke, Sinbad, Randy Travis, Sharon Stone, Sir Brian May, Loretta Lynn, Tim Curry.

In December of 2024 we learned about actor comedian Jamie Foxx and his stroke experience that he shared on a Netflix special. His humor and story reminded me of my humor approach and advice to dealing with the stroke experience.

In the YouTube universe there is a channel called World According to Briggs with 1.24M subscribers where Briggs provides an entertaining top ten list on a variety of topics. In October 2024, Briggs shared his stroke experience on his channel.

Staying Busy

I mentioned earlier about staying busy, and that would be one of the must-do's I strongly suggest. Staying both physically and mentally busy will benefit you. We must make physical activity and exercise part of our day in order to prevent spasticity from worsening. Staying mentally busy keeps our cognitive abilities from declining. I was able to continue teaching in an online environment. I also did a lot of writing; in addition to writing this book, I wrote a ten-part mystery book series called *Farmerville*.

My point here is to stay busy and not allow yourself to decline. You may not be a writer or teacher, but you can find things to do that do not include sitting on a couch. Keep busy, learn and do new things, and "Don't let those bad days win."

CLOSING THOUGHTS

This is not the end. Life goes on and continues forward with a positive attitude and approach to the path that life takes us on.

Physical limitations are not limits.

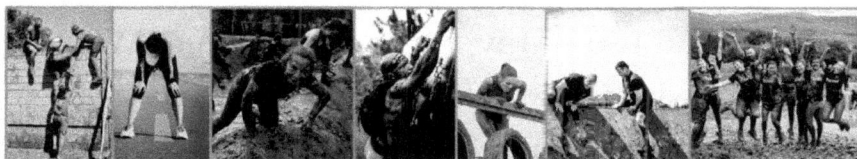

Navigate The Obstacles

Limitations are not limits, they are only obstacles we learn to navigate, to embrace, and to not let them win. It's like taking a detour to arrive at the same destination; you'll still get to where you're going, it's up to you how you get there.

When you started this book, the question I asked was, "Is this book for you?" I hope that this was the book for you and was and will be helpful to you as you navigate through the various stages of recovery, rehabilitation, and moving forward in your recovery. I've worked on this book for two and a half years, writing, editing, writing again, and editing again. I've experienced a variety of positives, slowdowns, setbacks, and experiences that ultimately provided you with some positive guidance, inspiration, and a sense of what to expect as you navigate through your recovery.

I had a stroke and spent a week in ICU, three weeks in a rehab hospital, and 10 months at outpatient therapy. I have damage to my left arm and leg, but putting the negatives aside, I can walk with a cane and have limited use of my left arm and hand. Whatever the task or destination, I take a detour to navigate my way to it and find success, and you will too.

There's no question that you'll find that I did not cover everything, or maybe I covered too much, but hopefully you will find what I've provided is beneficial.

I'll encourage you to not let the bad days win, don't quit, keep a positive attitude, and as Mr. Spock said, "Live long and prosper."

My plans are to be an advocate for stroke victims, maintaining a website, Facebook page, and YouTube channel, so if you are interested, I invite you to join me.

"Live long and prosper."

MOTIVATIONAL & INSPIRING THOUGHTS AND QUOTES

The little things will make a difference.

Repetition, Repetition, Repetition!

Keep your brain busy.

Don't let depression get ahold of you.

Don't quit!

Don't resist change.

*It's not just recovery and rehabilitation,
it's the rest of your life.*

*Grimace with a smile and chuckle when it
hurts.*

Stroke-surviving death dodger
You are not the only victim.
The emotions are coming.
Don't let depression get ahold of you.
Don't quit!
Don't make the mistake of slowing down!
Retrain your brain.
Set yourself up for success—not failure.
There it is: A goal to go rucking again.
Don't come up with reasons why you can't. Come up with the reasons why you can.
Don't let the bad days win.
Don't be upset by the results you didn't get from the work you did not do.
Visualize your goals.
Physical limitations are not limits.
Don't quit and don't *give up!*
Live long and prosper.

RESOURCES & REFERENCES
Resources

In addition to the list below, the power of a Google or internet search can provide countless other resources that may include local resources in your area.

American Stroke Association: https://www.stroke.org/

American Stroke Foundation: https://americanstroke.org/

Stroke Onward: https://strokeonward.org/stlouis/

Stroke Recovery Timeline, Johns Hopkins Medicine:
https://www.hopkinsmedicine.org/health/conditions-and-diseases/stroke/stroke-recovery-timeline

Stroke Resource Library: For Patients and Caregivers, American Stroke Association:
https://www.stroke.org/en/help-and-support/resource-library

Stroke: Resources for Caregiver & Survivors, SSMHealth:
https://www.ssmhealth.com/neurosciences/stroke/resources-for-caregivers-survivors

The Stroke Foundation: https://thestrokefoundation.org/
The Stroke Network: Online Stroke Support and
Information Resources: https://strokenetwork.org/

References

Bindawas, Saad M., and Vishal S. Vennu, "Stroke
rehabilitation: A call to action in Saudi Arabia,"
NeuroSciences, October 2016,
https://pmc.ncbi.nlm.nih.gov/articles/PMC5224426/

Klein AW, Mantell A. Electromyographic guidance in
injecting botulinum toxin. Dermatol Surg. 1998
Nov;24(11):1184-6. doi: 10.1111/j.1524-
4725.1998.tb04096.x. PMID: 9834737

Lee, June, "How to manage hand spasticity – Hand splint
after stroke," Neofect, July 14, 2021,
https://www.neofect.com/us/blog/how-to-manage-
hand-spasticity-after-stroke

Tobias, Tara, "How do you fix a heavy leg," Orlando
Neuro Therapy, Oct. 2, 2019,
https://orlandoneurotherapy.com/stroke/heavy-leg-
exercise/

"What is Stroke?" UTMB Health, accessed Nov. 21, 2024,
https://www.utmbhealth.com/services/neurology/proc
edures-conditions/stroke/what-is-stroke

ABOUT MARTY

Marty Martin (Warren, Pop Pop, Dr. Martin) grew up in New York City where he attended St. Stephens of Hungary elementary school and Power Memorial Academy high school. He joined the Army in 1975 where he met his wife Debbie, and they had three great kids and did some travels around the world. During his 21 years in the Army, he was in the infantry, military police and caught the bug to jump out of perfectly good airplanes and also volunteered for Special Forces *(Green Berets)*.

After he retired from the Army in 1996 he transitioned to business, working for Domino's Pizza Corporation and later was a Domino's franchise business owner. He earned his Ph.D. in Business Administration and Organizational Leadership from North Central University and his MBA from the

University of Michigan *(Go Blue)*. Marty transitioned to teaching at Norwich University and Bryan University in Springfield Missouri where he is the Business Program Chair and lives with his wife, Debbie Kay, in St. Louis Missouri.

Marty is a member of numerous writing organizations and is President of the Missouri Writers' Guild and past President of the St. Louis Publishers Association. He has a debut award winning novel titled "Forgotten Soldiers: What Happened to Jacob Walden." As a Grandparent he has a an award winning Children's book series based on his experiences with his grandchildren "Adventures with Pop Pop". Marty's latest fiction writing is the Mystery Thriller Series titled "Farmerville."

Surviving the Stroke Website

Marty Martin Website

Marty Martin Facebook

www.ingramcontent.com/pod-product-compliance
Lightning Source LLC
Chambersburg PA
CBHW070118030426
42335CB00016B/2193